The Clinician's Guide to Swallowing Fluoroscopy

Peter C. Belafsky • Maggie A. Kuhn

The Clinician's Guide to Swallowing Fluoroscopy

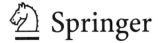
Springer

Peter C. Belafsky
Center for Voice and Swallowing
Department of Otolaryngology Head and
Neck Surgery
University of California, Davis
School of Medicine
Department of Medicine and Epidemiology
University of California, Davis School of
Veterinary Medicine
Sacramento, CA
USA

Maggie A. Kuhn
Center for Voice and Swallowing
Department of Otolaryngology Head
and Neck Surgery
University of California, Davis School
of Medicine
Sacramento, CA
USA

ISBN 978-1-4939-1108-0   ISBN 978-1-4939-1109-7 (eBook)
DOI 10.1007/978-1-4939-1109-7
Springer New York Heidelberg Dordrecht London

Library of Congress Control Number: 2014940394

Printed on acid-free paper

Springer is part of Springer Science+Business Media (www.springer.com)

Contents

Chapter 1
Radiation Safety

The dysphagia clinician must possess a thorough understanding of radiation safety in order to ensure the well being of both patients and fluoroscopists. An advanced knowledge of the tenants of appropriate radiation use is paramount for all swallowing clinicians conducting videofluoroscopic swallow studies (VFSS).

Ionizing radiation has the potential to injure individuals directly (somatic effects) as well as indirectly through the production of undesirable consequences in future generations (genetic effects). Somatic effects include injuries to superficial tissues, damage to a developing fetus, cataract formation, and cancer induction. Approximately 1–2% of all cancers are thought to result from exposure to radiation during medical imaging or therapy. In 2011, Berrington de Gonzalez estimated a lifetime cancer risk of 4–7 per 1,000 men and 6–13 per 1,000 women in the UK who undergo routine screening radiographic evaluations. The most common radiation-induced cancers include breast, thyroid, hematopoietic, lung, gastrointestinal, and bone. Genetic or inherited effects of radiation are a consequence of excessive gonadal exposure and manifest generations after the original radiation damage occurs. The radiation dose will vary among patient's tissues during VFSS and the unique susceptibility of individual tissues to the effects of ionizing radiation also differs. Where the head, neck, chest, and upper abdomen are concerned, particularly vulnerable areas include the eyes (lens), skin, thyroid, and bone marrow.

Limiting unnecessary radiation exposure begins with careful patient selection. The indication for VFSS should warrant the patient's exposure to radiation that the study will require. Common indications include dysphagia, odynophagia, aspiration, chronic cough, and postoperative evaluation. If a clinical question may be answered with another, non-radiographic diagnostic procedure, the potential advantages, limitations, and adverse effects of each should be weighed. For most clinical presentations of dysphagia, the VFSS and the videofluoroscopic esophagram (VFE) are considered the gold standard and medically acceptable diagnostic tools to evaluate swallow function. Modalities that do not employ radiation include the clinical or bedside swallow evaluation, flexible endoscopic examination of swallowing (FEES), high-resolution manometry, esophagoscopy, and guided observation of swallowing in the esophagus (GOOSE). These may be considered when clinically

P. C. Belafsky, M. A. Kuhn, *The Clinician's Guide to Swallowing Fluoroscopy,*
DOI 10.1007/978-1-4939-1109-7_1, © Springer Science+Business Media New York 2014

Table 1.1 Comparison of radiation doses

Source	Dose (mSv)
Chest X-ray	0.01
Trans-Atlantic flight	0.04
Videofluoroscopic swallow study	0.04–1.00
CT scan (head)	2
Annual background radiation	3
CT scan (abdominal)	5

CT computed tomography

Table 1.2 Radiation safety checklist

Assess chance of pregnancy	☐
Dosimetry badge	☐
Lead apron for clinician	☐
Thyroid shield for clinician	☐
Protective glasses for clinician	☐
Protective gloves for clinician	☐
Proper patient positioning in radiation field	☐
Proper collimation	☐
Gonad shield for patient	☐
Remove jewelry in radiation field of view	☐
Lights dimmed in fluoroscopy suite	☐

appropriate or when evaluating vulnerable populations such as children, women of reproductive age, and pregnant women.

Several units of measure are used to denote radiation amount and include gray, rads, and seiverts (Sv). When considering radiation's effect on human tissues, the Sv is generally preferred and employed as it has been normalized for various tissue effects of radiation. During a typical VFSS, radiation doses of up to 1 mSv may be delivered though many studies achieve a far lower dose, even as little as 0.04 mSv. This dose is understandably higher than that experienced during a single chest X-ray but is in well below the exposure received during a computed tomography (CT) scan. Table 1.1 compares radiation doses from various sources.

Organizations overseeing and governing the population's radiation exposure include the National Council for Radiation Protection (NCRP) and the International Atomic Energy Association (IAEA). These bodies assert that there is no acceptably safe radiation dose threshold and recommend adhering to the "as low as reasonable achievable" (ALARA) principle. This implies that any dose of radiation may result in an undesirable effect though this effect may be too slight to measure. Therefore, in order to reduce the risk to patients and practitioners, radiation doses should be kept as low as reasonably achievable. Radiation monitoring devices (radiation dosimeter) are worn by individuals who may receive doses of ionizing radiation that exceed 10% of the annual applicable allowable limit, and this includes clinicians who perform VFSS. The total effective dose equivalent (TEDA) is 0.05 Sv and represents the annual whole-body occupational external radiation limit. Women who are pregnant must declare so and may wear a fetal dosimetry badge. A pregnant woman's annual allowable ionizing radiation limit is 1 mSv. A radiation safety checklist is presented in Table 1.2.

Fig. 1.1 Satisfactory preparation and positioning for VFSS with appropriate radiation precautions observed

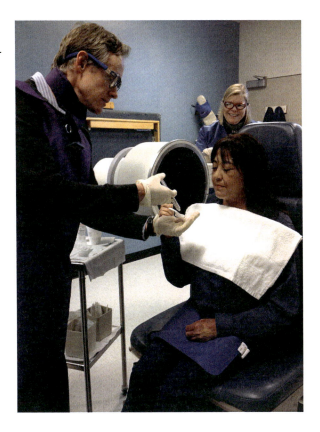

Factors directly influencing the amount of radiation delivered to a patient include X-ray tube characteristics of peak voltage (kVp), milliamperage (mA), collimation, and filtration. Additionally, exposure time, image field size, and distance of source to patient and to detector are directly related to the total radiation dose.

Modern fluoroscopy equipment offers a number of features meant to decrease radiation dose including collimation to the area of clinical interest, last frame hold, automatic kVp adjustment, image intensifier mode, and adjustable frame rates. These parameters should be set to reduce patient exposures while preserving the integrity of the VFSS. Frame rates should not be acquired below 30 frames per second (fps) as slower rates would significantly reduce the study's sensitivity and the clinician's ability to detect pathologic subtleties. All fluoroscopic swallowing examinations should be digitally recorded for later playback, which obviates the need to repeat sequences for real-time evaluation. Additionally, the fluoroscopic exposure switch must be a "dead-man" type, which terminates exposure when pressure is released. This is generally supplied in the form of a pedal.

Fluoroscopists and clinicians play a crucial role in preventing undue radiation exposure (Figs. 1.1 and 1.2). Firstly, they are responsible for determining the total radiation exposure time. This time should be adequate to obtain valuable clinical

Fig. 1.2 Unsatisfactory preparation and positioning for VFSS. *A* gonad shielding missing; *B* subject too close to emission source; *C* fluoroscopist missing thyroid shield; *D* clinician missing thyroid shield and dosimetry badge; *E* hand is in path of radiation and is ungloved; *F* no protective eye wear; *G* bright light illuminating fluoroscopy suite should be turned off

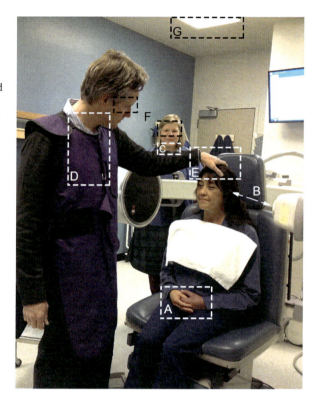

information but not excessive. Methodical protocols are useful to achieve this efficiency and are discussed further in Chaps. 2 and 3. Fluoroscopy time should be no longer than 5 min and, in our center, averages less than 3 min. Patients should be positioned such that the area of clinical interest is in the center of the collimated radiation field before fluoroscopy is activated. Subjects should also be instructed to remain still as unnecessary motion will diminish the image quality.

The fluoroscopist or clinician must also ensure the use of recommended and appropriate shielding. For the patient, a gonad shield of at least 0.5 mm lead equivalent is required and placed over the pelvis. The fluoroscopist must wear a lead apron of at least 0.25 mm lead equivalent, a protective thyroid collar, and a personnel monitoring device (dosimetry badge). Additional available protective devices include leaded glasses and gloves. Other individuals present during the fluoroscopic study such as clinicians or family members should don lead aprons and thyroid protection collars. The patient should be positioned as closely as possible to the detector while located at least 12 in., and ideally 18 in., from the emission source. Clinicians should remain at least 5 ft from the source and ideally behind a screen or curtain if available. Turning off the lights in the fluoroscopy suite will improve image contrast and afford the use of lower radiation doses. The image receptor quality should be maximized by updating to contemporary devices and radiation scatter should be reduced by removing objects from the emission beam path.

Fluoroscopic swallow studies are an essential component of the swallowing clinician's diagnostic repertoire but their safe practice demands reliable adherence to radiation safety protocols. When these appropriate measures are taken, negative consequences to both the subject and practitioner are acceptably reduced.

Suggested Reading

Belafsky PC, Rees CJ. Functional oesophagoscopy: endoscopic evaluation of the oesophageal phase of deglutition. J Laryngol Otol. 2009 Sept;123(9):1031–4.

Berrington de Gonzalez A. Estimates of potential risk of radiation-related cancer from screening in the UK. J Med Screen. 2011;18(4):163–4.

California Department of Health Services. Syllabus on fluoroscopy radiation protection. 6th ed.

Langmore SE, Schatz K, Olsen N. Fiberoptic endoscopic examination of swallowing safety: a new procedure. Dysphagia. 1988;2(4):216–9.

Martin-Harris B, Logemann JA, McMahon S, Schleicher M, Sandidge J. Clinical utility of the modified barium swallow. Dysphagia. 2000 Summer;15(3):136–41.

McCullough GH, Rosenbek JC, Wertz RT, McCoy S, Mann G, McCullough K. Utility of clinical swallowing examination measures for detecting aspiration post-stroke. J Speech Lang Hear Res. 2005 Dec;48(6):1280–93.

Pandolfino JE, Ghosh SK, Rice J, Clarke JO, Kwiatek MA, Kahrilas PJ. Classifying esophageal motility by pressure topography characteristics: a study of 400 patients and 75 controls. Am J Gastroenterol. 2008 Jan;103(1):27–37.

Smith-Bindman R, Lipson J, Marcus R, Kim KP, Mahesh M, Gould R et al. Radiation dose associated with common computed tomography examinations and the associated lifetime attributable risk of cancer. Arch Intern Med. 2009 Dec 14;169(22):2078–86.

Chapter 2
The Videofluoroscopic Swallow Study Technique and Protocol

The videofluoroscopic swallow study (VFSS) is the current gold standard for the diagnosis and management of oropharyngeal dysphagia. It provides a comprehensive evaluation of the oral, palatal, pharyngeal, and pharyngoesophageal segments of deglutition. Other terms to describe a radiographic swallow study include the modified barium swallow, the dynamic swallow study, and the cookie swallow. The American Speech-Language-Hearing Association (ASHA) routinely uses the terminology "videofluoroscopic swallow study," and it will likewise be used to refer to this investigation throughout this text. The VFSS does not uniformly include an evaluation of the esophageal phase of deglutition. The esophageal portion of the comprehensive swallow study will be referred to as the videofluoroscopic esophagram (VFE—Chap. 3).

Various techniques have been described to perform the VFSS. Methods differ from institution to institution; variables include the type, consistency, and quantity of contrast agent used. The swallowing clinician must be aware that variation exists among radiographic technique, equipment used, radiologic view, study capture rate, and patient position. Each of these factors has a significant contribution to the information acquired during the investigation. In order to reliably compare studies between patients and within patients pre- and post-intervention, it is essential to perform every investigation in a standardized and systematic manner. Precise and reproducible VFSS interpretation depends on this methodological approach. The protocol we use has been refined over 30 years of practice at our Center and is described in detail below.

We perform all of our studies using a properly collimated OEC Medical Systems mobile 9800 Radiographic/Fluoroscopic unit (OEC Medical Systems, Salt Lake City, UT) that provides 63 kV, 1.2 mA-type output for the full field-of-view mode (12-in. input phosphor diameter). We prefer the mobility of the C-arm to fixed fluoroscopic units (Fig. 2.1). The orbital rotation of the C-arm affords flexibility and provides the ability to study patients of various sizes at diverse angles and image projections. All studies are performed in a lead-lined room by a licensed radiology technician and speech language pathologist (SLP) and are later reviewed by a physician licensed in fluoroscopy from the Radiologic Health Branch (RHB) of the California Food, Drug, and Radiation Safety Division of the Department of Public

P. C. Belafsky, M. A. Kuhn, *The Clinician's Guide to Swallowing Fluoroscopy*,
DOI 10.1007/978-1-4939-1109-7_2, © Springer Science+Business Media New York 2014

Fig. 2.1 Positioning of the
C-arm fluoroscopic unit during examination of a patient
in the lateral fluoroscopic
view. There is a disk of
known diameter taped under
the chin, a towel protecting
the clothing from spilled
barium, and a lead apron
shielding the reproductive
organs

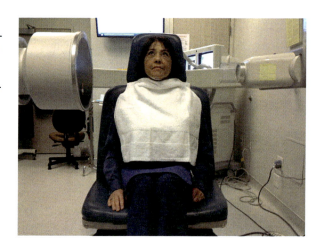

Health. The studies are digitally recorded on nStream G3 HD/SD (Image Stream
Medical Inc., Littleton, MA) at 30 frames per second (fps) for later slow motion
playback and analysis. The nStream system is integrated with the electronic medical
record (Epic Systems, Verona, Wisconsin) and can be accessed from any computer
with an internet connection.

The ability to record the studies at 30 fps and review in a frame-by-frame manner is essential for precise interpretation and analysis. Studies obtained at capture
rates less than 30 fps may miss significant pathology. All examinations are reviewed
weekly during an interdisciplinary panel that includes SLPs, nurses, physicians,
students, and dietitians.

Patients are weighed, measured, and given the validated ten-item Eating Assessment Tool (EAT-10) prior to the administration of barium and the results are documented in the EMR (Fig. 2.2). The height and weight afford calculation of the BMI,
which assists with the assessment of nutritional status. The association of patient
symptoms captured by the EAT-10 with VFSS findings provides essential information to assist the clinician with the development of a comprehensive treatment
plan. The EAT-10 documents the level of baseline disability and is instrumental in
monitoring treatment efficacy.

We use a 60 % weight/volume (w/v) ratio of barium sulfate (Fig. 2.3; EZpaque,
Westbury, NJ). This contrast agent has the rheological properties of a nectar thick
liquid. The use of a nectar thick liquid for the VFSS has advantages and limitations.
Higher density barium formulations (nectar and honey thick) are more viscous. The
increased viscosity and subsequent mucosal adherence provides better visualization of subtle pathology such as webs, rings, and cricopharyngeus muscle bars that
may otherwise be missed. The higher density barium is also more radiopaque and
is easier to visualize under fluoroscopy. Less dense agents that behave like a thin
liquid do not provide the anatomic detail nor possess the mucosal adherence of the
thicker formulations. Although our protocol does not routinely utilize less dense,
thinner barium for these reasons, we will, on occasion, dilute the suspension by

Eating Assessment Tool (EAT-10)
Circle the appropriate response

To what extent are the following scenarios problematic for you?	0 = No problem 4 = Severe problem				
1. My swallowing problem has caused me to lose weight.	0	1	2	3	4
2. My swallowing problem interferes with my ability to go out for meals.	0	1	2	3	4
3. Swallowing liquids takes extra effort.	0	1	2	3	4
4. Swallowing solids takes extra effort.	0	1	2	3	4
5. Swallowing pills takes extra effort.	0	1	2	3	4
6. Swallowing is painful.	0	1	2	3	4
7. The pleasure of eating is affected by my swallowing.	0	1	2	3	4
8. When I swallow food sticks in my throat.	0	1	2	3	4
9. I cough when I eat.	0	1	2	3	4
10. Swallowing is stressful.	0	1	2	3	4
				Total EAT-10	

Fig. 2.2 The ten-item Eating Assessment Tool (EAT-10)

Fig. 2.3 Sixty percent
weight/volume ratio of
barium sulfate (EZpaque,
Westbury, NJ)

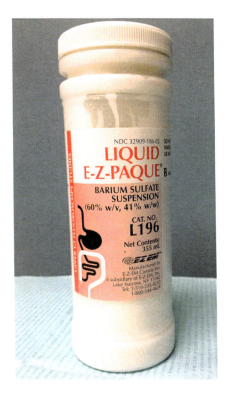

Fig. 2.4 Boundaries of the lateral fluoroscopic view (*1* lips, *2* nasopharynx, *3* cervical spine, *4* cervical esophagus). There is also an obstructing cricopharyngeus muscle bar (*red asterisk*) and a dilated pharynx (*red arrowheads*)

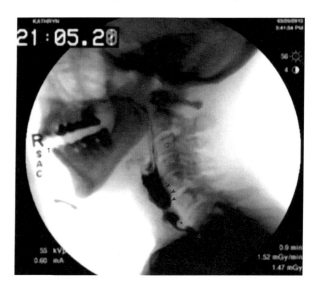

50 % using water. Patients at risk of aspirating thin liquids will have an increased likelihood of aspirating the thinner barium formulation. The information acquired from the thinner, less dense formulation may assist with treatment recommendations but it will also have direct implications on study analysis. All of the normative data for the objective fluoroscopic measures that we use (Chap. 7) are based on use of the 60 % w/v barium concentration. Altering the density of the barium will have a direct effect on deglutitive measures such as pharyngeal transit time and opening. This alteration will make the interpretation of objective fluoroscopic measures inaccurate. For this reason, we perform the majority of our VFSSs with the 60 % w/v formulation. It is essential that the clinician take the density of the barium into consideration when performing and analyzing these investigations. A comprehensive investigation of the benefits and limitations of precise barium formulations has not been conducted and warrants future study. Our experience suggests that the 60 % w/v formulation provides a balance between the desired rheology and the ability to provide optimal anatomic detail.

The patient is positioned in an examination chair with the fluoroscopy unit in the lateral position. The patient head position is neutral and facing forward (Fig. 2.1). Clothing, jewelry, and other artifacts that may interfere with the fluoroscopic image are removed and stored. A lead apron is placed over the patient's pelvic region to protect the reproductive organs and a towel is draped over the shoulders and lap to prevent drips of barium from getting on patient clothing. A radiopaque disk of known diameter (19 mm) is secured to the patient's chin with tape to allow for later calibration during the on screen calculation of objective fluoroscopic swallow measures (Chap. 7). The boundaries of the fluoroscopy field in the lateral view are the lips anteriorly, nasopharynx superiorly, cervical spine posteriorly, and cervical esophagus inferiorly (Fig. 2.4). The boundaries of the fluoroscopy field in the anterior-posterior (AP) view are the walls of the pharynx laterally, the nasopharynx

Fig. 2.5 Boundaries of the anterior-posterior fluoroscopic view (*1* lateral pharyngeal walls, *2* nasopharynx, *3* cervical esophagus)

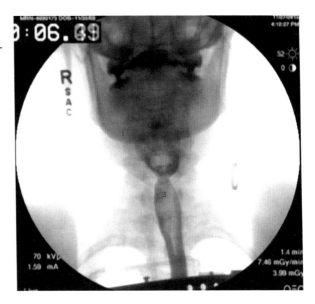

superiorly, and the cervical esophagus inferiorly (Fig. 2.5). The patient is positioned upright with the spine perpendicular and the chin parallel to the floor. A standardized position is essential. Subtle variations in head tilt or position may alter swallowing biomechanics and are to be avoided unless specific maneuvers are being tested.

The study protocol proceeds in a stepwise fashion (Table 2.1). If the initial barium administration does not pose a threat to patient safety, the study proceeds to the next bolus size without a change in instruction. If swallowing function is determined to be hazardous, the protocol is modified to enhance patient safety. Compensatory maneuvers such as a chin tuck, head turn, or breath hold may be utilized. These strategies will alter swallowing biomechanics and must be noted during the interpretation of the study. If the maneuvers are unsuccessful and the further administration of barium poses too great a threat to patient safety, the study is terminated. The harm from potential barium aspiration must be weighed against the need to obtain quality information that will lead to improved patient health.

Patients are administered liquid barium boluses in precise aliquots of 1, 3, and 20 ml in the lateral fluoroscopic view. The barium is administered by syringe for the 1 and 3 ml boluses and by graduated medicine cup for the 20 ml bolus. For each bolus, the patient is instructed to hold the bolus in the oral cavity and wait. The patient is then instructed to, "swallow it all at once." Following the liquid barium, the patient is administered a 3 ml 60% w/w barium paste bolus (E-Z-Paste; E-Z-EM, Inc.). A 60 ml liquid barium bolus is then administered by sequential straw drinking. The patient is instructed to place the straw in their mouth and drink the barium as fast as they can. The radiopaque disk is moved to a location at the level of the UES and the patient is positioned in the AP view. Liquid barium boluses of 3 and 20 ml, and a 13 mm barium tablet (Merry X-Ray Corp., San Diego, CA) are administered.

Table 2.1 VFSS protocol

Lateral fluoroscopic view
1 ml 60% w/v liquid barium
3 ml 60% w/v liquid barium
20 ml 60% w/v liquid barium
3 ml 60% w/w barium paste
60 ml 60% w/v liquid barium sequential straw task
Anterior–posterior fluoroscopic view
3 ml 60% w/v liquid barium
20 ml 60% w/v liquid barium
13 mm barium tablet

VFSS videofluoroscopic swallow study

The AP fluoroscopic view provides important clinical information regarding the laterality of bolus flow and pharyngeal residue that cannot be obtained from the lateral projection. It also provides an important assessment of AP opening. Normative data on AP opening are available and diminished opening identifies pathology such as a stenosis or web that may be missed on the lateral study. The AP view also provides important information regarding the dimensions and location of pharyngeal (pulsion), pharyngoesophageal (Zenker), and cervical esophageal (traction) diverticuli (Fig. 2.5).

The patient is again returned to the lateral position. Speech tasks are performed to evaluate palatal competence. The patient is asked to say a repeated "k" and then "ka" to evaluate lingual-palatal and velopharyngeal competence. The patient may be asked to cough and spit to evaluate the effectiveness of clearing penetrated or aspirated barium. Asking the patient to blow against resistance may also be performed to assess asymmetries in pharyngeal wall tone.

If the etiology of the patients swallowing function is not revealed at the completion of the protocol, the patient may be administered a thin liquid bolus by diluting the barium with 50% water. Patient-specific dysphagia complaints such as certain swallowing positions or particular foods may be studied after completion of the systematic protocol. If protective maneuvers or positioning strategies have not been evaluated then they are performed before the study is complete. Total fluoroscopy time is limited to 3 min or less.

Suggested Reading

Belafsky PC, Mouadeb DA, Rees CJ, Pryor JC, Postma GN, Allen J, Leonard RJ. Validity and reliability of the Eating Assessment Tool (EAT-10). Ann Otol Rhinol Laryngol. 2008 Dec;117(12):919–24.

Fink TA, Ross JB. Are we testing a true thin liquid? Dysphagia. 2009 Sep;24(3):285–9.

Kendall KA, Leonard RJ, McKenzie S. Airway protection: evaluation with videofluoroscopy. Dysphagia. 2004 Spring;19(2):65–70.

Kendall KA, Leonard RJ, McKenzie SW. Accommodation to changes in bolus viscosity in normal deglutition: a videofluoroscopic study. Ann Otol Rhinol Laryngol. 2001 Nov;110(11):1059–65.

Leonard RJ, Kendall KA, McKenzie S, Gonçalves MI, Walker A. Structural displacements in normal swallowing: a videofluoroscopic study. Dysphagia. 2000 Summer;15(3):146–52.

Leonard R, Kendall C, editors. Dysphagia assessment and treatment planning: a team approach. 2nd edn. San Diego: Plural Publishing; 2007.

Shaker R, Belafsky PC, Postma GN, Easterling C, editors. Principles of deglutition: a multidisciplinary text for swallowing and its disorders. New York: Springer; 2012.

Shaker R, Belafsky PC, Postma GN, Easterling C, editors. Manual of diagnostic and therapeutic techniques for disorders of deglutition. New York: Springer; 2012.

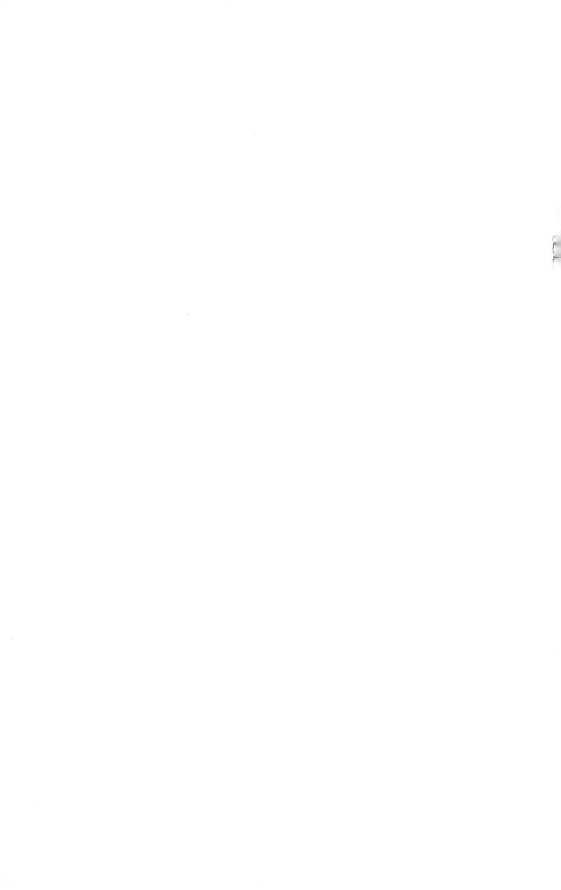

Chapter 3
The Videofluoroscopic Esophagram Technique and Protocol

One-third of individuals who localize the source of dysphagia to the cervical region will have an esophageal etiology for their swallowing dysfunction. It is as if the drainpipe is clogged down the line and all that the patient feels is the toilet overflowing. A healthy ambulatory patient with the chief complaint of solid food dysphagia will have an esophageal contribution to their swallowing dysfunction in nearly 60 % of cases. A thorough evaluation of the esophagus is essential in the comprehensive work-up of persons with dysphagia and an advanced understanding of the methodology and analysis of the videofluoroscopic esophagram (VFE) is fundamental for all swallowing clinicians.

Esophagography can evaluate both structural (webs, rings, strictures) and motility disorders of the esophagus. To reliably compare studies between patients and within patients pre- and post-intervention, it is essential to perform every VFE in a systematic manner. Precise and reproducible interpretation depends on this methodological approach. The protocol for esophagography we use has been refined over 30 years of practice at our center.

We differentiate the fluoroscopic evaluation of the esophagus into an esophageal screen (ES) and a comprehensive VFE. A comprehensive VFE is not feasible or necessary in all individuals. Limitations in clinical resources and personnel or patient factors such as physical restrictions in mobility or positioning may preclude the performance of a comprehensive esophageal examination. Oropharyngeal swallowing dysfunction may also limit the ability to safely consume enough barium by mouth to perform a thorough esophageal evaluation. These factors, in addition to the desire to limit patient radiation exposure, led to the development of an ES as an alternative to the comprehensive VFE when the clinical suspicion for esophageal pathology is limited. When compared to a comprehensive VFE as the gold standard, the sensitivity of the ES is 63 % and the specificity is 100 %. Thus, an abnormal ES may dictate future clinical management but a normal screen does rule out the presence of esophageal pathology. Because of the high prevalence of esophageal pathology, we advocate an ES in all patients who undergo a videofluoroscopic swallow study (VFSS) who are not scheduled to have a comprehensive VFE. Our speech and language pathology team routinely performs the ES as an adjunct to all VFSSs when the patient is not scheduled to undergo a comprehensive VFE. A comprehen-

P. C. Belafsky, M. A. Kuhn, *The Clinician's Guide to Swallowing Fluoroscopy.*
DOI 10.1007/978-1-4939-1109-7_3, © Springer Science+Business Media New York 2014

Table 3.1 Esophageal screen
protocol

| *Anterior–posterior fluoroscopic view* |
| 20 ml 60% w/v liquid barium |
| 13 mm barium tablet |

sive VFE is warranted in patients with a normal ES when there exists a high index of suspicion for esophageal pathology.

We use a 60% weight/volume (w/v) ratio of barium sulfate (EZpaque, Westbury, NJ) for all standard VFE examinations. This suspension has the rheological properties of a nectar thick liquid. There are benefits to using a diluted barium suspension that behaves more like a thin liquid. Altering the density of the barium affects the viscosity, rheological properties, and esophageal biomechanics required to transport the material into the stomach and must be considered during analysis. Diluted formulations of barium afford less anatomic detail but more closely approximate the desired rheological properties of a thin liquid. A comprehensive investigation of the benefits and limitations of precise barium formulations utilized during the ES and VFE has not been conducted and is warranted. Our experience suggests that the 60% w/v formulation provides a balance between the desired rheology and the ability to provide optimal anatomic detail.

If the presence of a pharyngeal or esophageal perforation is suspected, a water-soluble contrast medium such as Omnipaque (GE Healthcare Inc., Buckinghamshire, UK) or Gastrografin (Bracco Diagnostic Inc., Monroe Township, NJ) may be utilized. If barium extravasates into the mediastinum, it may persist for months and complicate the interpretation of future imaging studies or predispose to granuloma formation and mediastinitis. Barium also adheres to mucosal surfaces and may significantly complicate forthcoming endoscopy. The water-soluble contrast agents are rapidly resorbed and do not have these shortcomings. They are, however, less radiopaque and are less adherent than barium and small perforations may be missed in up to 50% of cases. In addition, the water-soluble agents may cause a chemical pneumonitis if aspirated. Barium, in comparison, is well tolerated in the lungs. For these reasons, we do not administer barium if endoscopy is imminent and we only administer water-soluble agents with caution and only in persons without a history of oropharyngeal dysphagia. In addition, we routinely administer barium if the water-soluble contrast fails to detect a leak. All studies are standardized and digitally recorded for later playback and interpretation.

All studies are captured and reviewed at 30 frames per second (fps). The use of spot films or studies recorded with lower capture rates significantly limits analysis and may result in missing subtle pathology such as transient webs or rings.

ES Technique

The ES (Table 3.1) is performed after completion of the oropharyngeal phase of the VFSS (Chap. 2). The patient is positioned on a chair in the anterior–posterior (AP) view. The patient is given a lead shield to protect the pelvic region. Clothing,

Fig. 3.1 Positioning for
seated anterior–posterior
esophagram. There is a disk
of known diameter taped to
the right side of the neck, a
towel protecting the clothing
from spilled barium, and
a lead apron shielding the
reproductive organs

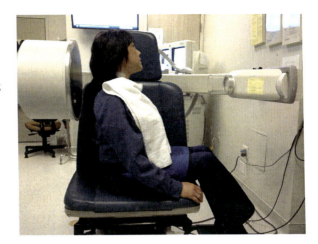

Fig. 3.2 Positioning for
standing anterior–posterior
esophagram

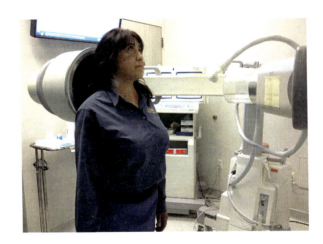

jewelry, or other artifacts obstructing the fluoroscopic field are removed. A towel
is draped over the shoulders and lap to prevent drips of barium on the patient's
clothing (Fig. 3.1). The study begins with the administration of a single bolus of
20 ml 60 % w/v liquid barium. The patient is instructed to swallow the entire bolus
in one hard swallow. Additional swallows per bolus must be avoided. Esophageal
peristalsis halts as soon as a pharyngeal swallow is initiated, and the occurrence of
multiple pharyngeal swallows results in deglutitive inhibition, which significantly
alters the evaluation of esophageal function. This is reinforced by saying, "swallow
hard and swallow once." The bolus is followed all the way from the oral cavity to
its entry into the stomach. To accommodate the speed of lowering the C-arm while
tracking the bolus in taller individuals, the patient is positioned standing with knees
slightly flexed and asked to hold the bolus in the mouth, then swallow all at once
and straighten the knees to achieve full standing height. Screening during this maneuver follows the bolus from the oral cavity, down the entire length of the esophagus to the stomach (Fig. 3.2). The bolus is timed from the initiation of the swallow

until its entry into the esophagus. Normal esophageal peristalsis is approximately 2 cm/s, so the bolus should be cleared from a 25 cm esophagus in less than 15 s. Barium remaining in the esophagus after 15 s suggests the presence of esophageal pathology (ineffective motility, web, stricture, neoplasm, or other). After the administration of the 20 ml bolus in the AP view, the patient is given a 13 mm barium tablet (Merry X-Ray Corp., San Diego, CA). The tablet helps to identify a site of obstruction by revealing a lumen patency less than 13 mm and helps the examiner gauge the diameter of an obstructed lumen. The transit of the tablet is recorded under real-time fluoroscopy until it has entered the stomach. If there is significant delay in the passage of the tablet, the fluoroscopy is intermittently turned off to limit radiation exposure. The esophagus is evaluated every 60 s until the passage of the tablet or bolus or until 5 min has elapsed. The addition of the barium tablet to the ES increases the sensitivity of the examination to nearly 75 %. Total fluoroscopy time is limited to 30 s. If the site of dysphagia is still undetermined at the end of the ES, consideration is given to carrying out a comprehensive VFE.

Comprehensive VFE Technique

The patient is first evaluated upright in the AP view similar to the ES. We prefer the upright position for the initial swallows in order to evaluate the esophagus in a natural eating position with the benefit of gravity. The patient is positioned on a chair in the AP view (Fig. 3.1). The patient is given a lead shield to protect the pelvic region and obstructing clothing and jewelry are removed. A towel is draped over the shoulders and lap to prevent drips of barium on the patient's clothing. The patient is then given 20 ml of 60 % w/v liquid barium to consume via a cup without a straw. The patient is instructed to take the largest sip comfortable from the cup and consume the barium with one swallow. Initiating a second swallow will arrest and reinitiate esophageal peristalsis, affecting the evaluation of esophageal body motility (deglutitive inhibition). The patient is instructed to "swallow hard and swallow once." The bolus is followed from the oral cavity until it enters the stomach. Once the barium has cleared the entire esophagus, the patient is given a cup with 10 ml of effervescent crystals (EZ-Gas II; E-Z-EM, Lake Success, NY) and 10 ml of water and asked to drink rapidly. A second 20 ml barium bolus with identical instructions is then administered. Collapsed and partially collapsed mucosal relief views are obtained. Once the barium has cleared the esophagus, the patient is given a 2 oz cup of water and asked to swallow a 13 mm barium tablet. The tablet helps to identify a site of obstruction with a lumen size less than 13 mm. The examination is recorded under real-time fluoroscopy at 30 fps until the tablet has entered the stomach. If there is significant delay in the passage of the barium bolus or tablet, the fluoroscopy is intermittently turned off to limit radiation exposure. The esophagus is evaluated every 60 s until the passage of the tablet or bolus or until 5 min has elapsed.

Fig. 3.3 Positioning for right anterior oblique (RAO) esophageal view. The lead apron (*red arrow*) is placed between the patient and the fluoroscopy table

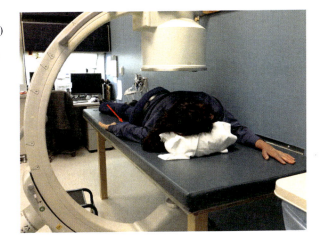

The patient is then placed recumbent on a table to acheive the right anterior oblique (RAO) projection. This position eliminates the benefit of gravity and helps identify esophageal dysmotility. The patient is placed chest down and turned to the left and instructed to rotate 40° so that the right anterior thorax is against the radiology table. The right arm is placed down at the side with the left arm flexed at the elbow and placed up by the head. The left knee is flexed and a bottle of liquid barium containing a straw is placed in their left hand (Fig. 3.3). The RAO position differentiates the esophagus from the spine and provides optimal orientation for the evaluation of esophageal anatomy and function. The patient is instructed to take the largest straw sip comfortable with similar instructions regarding the importance of a single swallow. The barium is followed from the oral cavity to its entry into the stomach. When the barium has cleared the esophagus, the patient is asked to gulp from the bottle with multiple swallows to maximally distend the esophagus. This sequential swallowing maneuver is essential to evaluate the esophagus for webs, rings, and hernias, particularly at the gastroesophageal junction (GEJ). Esophageal peristalsis should not be evaluated during the sequential swallow task because of deglutitive inhibition. If there is barium stasis in the transition zone of the esophagus (junction of proximal and middle third), the patient is asked to perform two dry swallows to relax the upper esophageal sphincter and evaluate for esophagopharyngeal reflux. If there is significant delay in the passage of the barium bolus, the fluoroscopy is intermittently turned off to limit radiation exposure. The esophagus is evaluated every 60 s with flash pedal-tap-only views until the passage of the bolus or until 5 min has elapsed.

The patient is then placed supine with their head on a pillow to simulate nocturnal positioning and provocative maneuvers are performed to evaluate for gastroesophageal reflux. The patient is asked to raise and hold their legs 6 in off of the fluoroscopy table for 10 s (Fig. 3.4). While in this position the patient is asked to perform a Valsalva maneuver and is subsequently asked to drink 80 ml of water to perform *the water siphon test*. The GEJ is visualized for the presence of gastroesophageal reflux

Fig. 3.4 Positioning for supine reflux provoking maneuvers. The patient is given water to sip via straw for the water siphon test

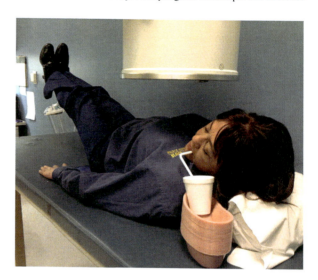

Table 3.2 Comprehensive videofluoroscopic esophagram protocol

Anterior–posterior fluoroscopic view
20 ml 60 % w/v liquid barium
10 ml effervescent crystals/10 ml water
20 ml 60 % w/v liquid barium
13 mm 60 % w/v liquid barium tablet/2 oz water
Right anterior oblique view
Largest single sip 60 % w/v liquid barium comfortable by straw sip
Largest sequential swallow task 60 % w/v liquid barium
Supine
Reflux provocation maneuvers
80 ml water siphon test

as the water passes into the stomach and relaxes the lower esophageal sphincter. The sensitivity of the comprehensive VFE in the diagnosis of gastroesophageal reflux disease is poor and may be as low as 20 %. The addition of the water siphon test significantly improves diagnostic sensitivity but at the expense of specificity. This completes the comprehensive VFE (Table 3.2). Total fluoroscopy time is limited to 2 min. The patient is advised to drink three 16-oz glasses of water throughout the remainder of the day to help clear the barium and prevent constipation.

Suggested Reading

Allen JE, White C, Leonard R, Belafsky PC. Comparison of esophageal findings on videofluoroscopy with full esophagram results. Head Neck. 2012 Feb;34(2):264–9.

Belafsky, P, Rees C. The role of esophagography in the evaluation of reflux disease. In: Johnston N, Toohill RJ, editors. Effects, diagnosis and management of extra-esophageal reflux. Hauppauge: Nova Science Publishers; 2010. pp. 89–96.

Buecker A, Wein BB, Neuerburg JM, Guenther RW. Esophageal perforation: comparison of use of aqueous and barium-containing contrast media. Radiology. 1997 Mar;2002(3):683–6.

Leonard R, Kendall C, editors. Dysphagia assessment and treatment planning: a team approach. 2nd edn. San Diego: Plural Publishing; 2007.

Shaker R, Belafsky PC, Postma GN, Easterling C, editors. Principles of deglutition: a multidisciplinary text for swallowing and its disorders. New York: Springer; 2012.

Shaker R, Belafsky PC, Postma GN, Easterling C, editors. Manual of diagnostic and therapeutic techniques for disorders of deglutition. New York: Springer; 2012.

Chapter 4
Normal Oral and Pharyngeal Phase Fluoroscopy

Deglutition is traditionally divided into four phases, beginning with oral preparatory and continuing through oral, pharyngeal, and esophageal phases. The traveling bolus is propelled by highly specialized anatomy that produces a series of chambers and valves which delineate the phases of swallowing. All phases may be captured during the videofluoroscopic swallow study (VFSS). The purpose of this chapter is to describe the expected fluoroscopic findings during the normal oral and pharyngeal phases of deglutition. The subsequent two chapters will explore normal pharyngoesophageal segment (PES) and esophageal fluoroscopy.

Normal Fluoroscopic Anatomy

The oral cavity consists of the lips, vestibule, bucal mucosa, mandibular and maxillary alveolar ridges with teeth, hard palate, anterior tongue and floor of mouth (Fig. 4.1). Extending from the base of the skull to the level of C6, the pharynx is divided into the nasopharynx, oropharynx, and hypopharynx (Fig. 4.2). The nasopharynx is not part of the alimentary tract but contains muscles that participate in swallowing by preventing movement of a food bolus into the nasal cavity. The oropharynx begins posterior to the oral cavity at the circumvallate papillae of the tongue and the junction of the hard and soft palates. It extends to the hyoid bone. The oropharynx is composed of the tongue base, palatoglossal and palatopharyngeal folds, palatine tonsils, lingual tonsil, lateral and posterior oropharyngeal walls, and vallecula (Fig. 4.1). The hypopharynx extends inferiorly from the hyoid bone and base of tongue to the esophageal inlet. It consists of paired piriform sinuses, postcricoid region, and posterior hypopharyngeal wall. The posterior and lateral walls of the pharynx are formed by the superior, middle, and inferior constrictor muscles.

Some oral and pharyngeal structures including the floor of mouth and lateral pharyngeal walls are not well delineated on fluoroscopy. However a number of osseous and soft tissue components are readily visible and may be reliably assessed

Fig. 4.1 A sagittal rendering of the oral cavity and oropharynx demonstrates normal anatomic structures. *CI* central incisor; *S* symphysis of mandible; *white arrowhead* floor of mouth; *white arrow* hard palate; *OT* oral tongue; *black arrowhead* soft palate; *black arrow* palatine tonsil; *bracket* base of tongue (Used with permission from Corey AS, Hudgins PA. Radiographic imaging of human papillomavirus related carcinomas of the oropharynx. Journal of Head and Neck Pathology. 2012 Jul; 6 (1): 25-40.)

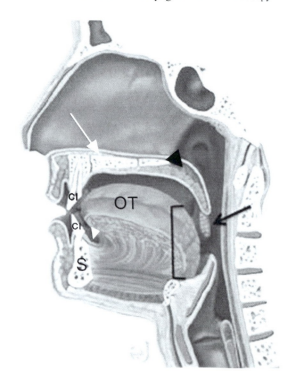

with the VFSS (Fig. 4.3). The mandible and maxilla with their associated teeth surround the visible fluoroscopic oral cavity. The oral tongue is best visualized when a radiopaque bolus is in the mouth or is coated with contrast. The soft palate and its most inferior component, the uvula, are generally identifiable as is the tongue base. Posterior to the tongue base, the epiglottis is visible in the air-filled common aerodigestive tract and forms the posterior limit of the vallecula. The posterior portion of the pharyngeal constrictors apposes the cervical spine and easily is assessed.

Normal anatomic findings include an intact mandibular arch of adequate height with a full complement of healthy teeth. The oral tongue should fill the oral vestibule and the tongue base should be visible beyond the angle of the mandible though not obscuring the vallecula. A perfectly normal epiglottis is thin having a width less than 8 mm or 33 % of the width of C4 (Fig. 4.4). It also follows a slight cranial curvature. The posterior pharyngeal wall should have a near uniform thickness measuring approximately 0.30–0.40 cm between C2 and C3 (Fig. 4.4). Findings outside of these standards may be considered normal and include altered or replaced dentition, mandibular atrophy in the elderly, vallecular filling by the lingual tonsil, retroflexion of the epiglottis, and mild pharyngeal wall thickening particularly if over-lying a prior surgical site or spinal fusion plate. Abnormal fluoroscopic oral and pharyngeal anatomy will be reviewed in Chap. 9.

Fig. 4.2 A sagittal drawing demonstrating the three components of the pharynx. (Used with permission from Lee SH. Upper airway structure during development. In: Kheirandish-Gozal L, Gozal D, editors. Sleep disordered breathing in children. New York. Springer Science + Business Media, LLC; 2012)

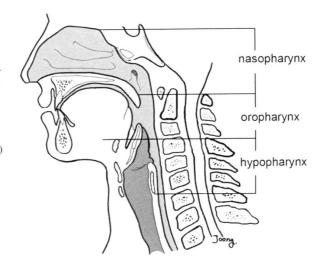

Fig. 4.3 Lateral fluoroscopic view demonstrating important oral and pharyngeal anatomy. *White dotted line* teeth; *black dashed line* mandible; *white arrowheads* oral tongue; *white dashed line* tongue base; *white arrows* soft palate; *black asterisk* nasopharynx; *black dotted line* epiglottis; *black arrowheads* posterior pharyngeal wall

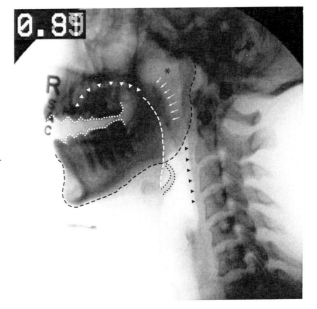

Normal Fluoroscopic Physiology

VFSS affords the unique ability to evaluate the posterior oral portion of deglutition, which remains hidden during clinical swallow evaluations and flexible endoscopic examination of swallowing (FEES). The VFSS is helpful in correlating clinical oral motor findings with bolus control.

Fig. 4.4 Lateral fluoroscopic view showing normal posterior pharyngeal wall (*black line*) and epiglottic thickness. An outline of the epiglottis (*grey dotted line*) has been superimposed to demonstrate that its width is less than 33 % of C4

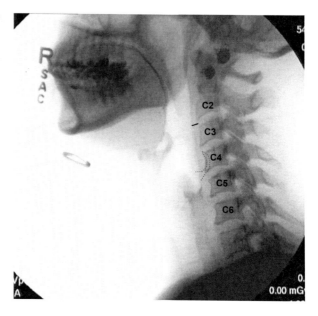

   The oral preparatory phase of deglutition is under voluntary control and includes mastication and bolus formation. Both are dependent on a moist, well-lubricated environment with healthy dentition and oral mucosa. Lip closure, mediated by the orbicularis oris muscle, is maintained throughout this phase, as well as the subsequent pharyngeal phase of swallowing. As such, normal oral and pharyngeal swallowing is accompanied by nasal breathing. Bolus preparation begins with containment by the labial valve or lips. This is readily assessed fluoroscopically as soon as the subject takes the bolus into their mouth (Fig. 4.5). Mastication is the mechanical processing of food that is ingested into the mouth and is accomplished by the masticatory apparatus including the teeth, jaw muscles, temporomandibular joint, tongue, lips, palate, and salivary glands. To limit radiation exposure, our center's protocol does not routinely include trials that require mastication as the integrity of this function can usually be discerned from the clinical oral motor examination.

   During oral bolus preparation the tensed soft palate and posterior tongue come together to form the linguapalatal valve, which contains the bolus within the oral cavity until it is ready to be released into the pharynx (Fig. 4.6). Incompetence of this valve may result in delayed initiation of swallow and premature entry of the bolus into the pharynx. Such abnormalities will be described in Chap. 9. Under normal circumstances, the linguapalatal valve opens and transmits the bolus completely into the oropharynx, which expands to accommodate the entering bolus. This is achieved by anterior motion of the tongue base and elasticity of the lateral pharyngeal walls.

   At the same time, the velopharyngeal valve closes through elevation and retraction of the soft palate, anterior movement of the posterior pharyngeal wall and medial movement of the lateral pharyngeal walls. The contribution of each component

Fig. 4.5 Lateral fluoroscopic view of labial containment (*black dotted lines*) of a 3 cc liquid barium bolus (*white dotted line*)

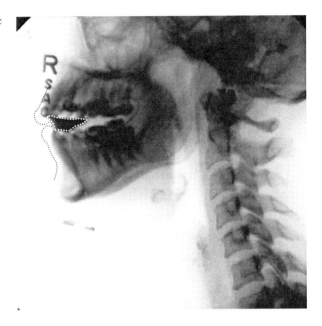

Fig. 4.6 Lateral fluoroscopic view of linguapalatal valve. The bolus (*white dotted line*) is kept in the oral cavity by tongue base (*black dashed line*) and soft palate (*white dashed line*) apposition

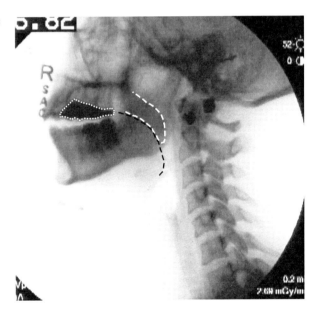

varies among individuals (Fig. 4.7). The competence of this valve protects against nasopharyngeal reflux of oropharyngeal contents and is essential to generate the pressure needed to propel the bolus through the oropharynx. This valve is also critical for articulation of plosives and fricatives. Clinical evaluation of velopharyngeal

Fig. 4.7 Lateral fluoroscopic view of velopharyngeal valve. The bolus (*white dotted line*) enters the oro-pharynx as the tongue base is brought anteriorly (*black dashed line*) and the soft palate (*white dashed line*) apposes the posterior pharyngeal wall (*black dotted line*). The valve protects against reflux into the nasopharynx (*black asterisk*)

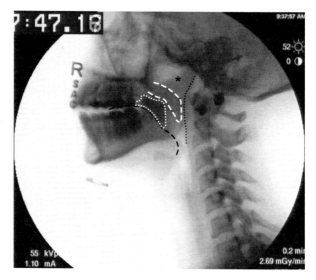

competence includes assessment of /s/, /p/, /b/, /d/, and /k/ sounds or a speech sample and observing for fog in a mirror place under a subjects nose during speech.

Contraction of the pharyngeal wall propels the bolus by providing the necessary pressure on its tail. On fluoroscopy, this is commonly referred to as the "pharyngeal wave." Opening of the PES depends, in part, on generation of adequate pharyngeal pressures (Fig. 4.8b, c). A surrogate measure of this pressure can be obtained from VFSS by calculating the pharyngeal constriction ratio (PCR), which is discussed in Chap. 7. Additionally, the anterior–superior motion during elevation of the hyo-laryngeal complex contributes to PES opening. This motion creates distal

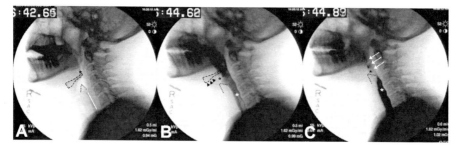

Fig. 4.8 Lateral fluoroscopic view of oral and pharyngeal bolus transit. As the bolus is propelled from the oral cavity to the oropharynx (**a**), the pharyngoesophageal segment (PES, *solid white line*) is closed and the hyoid bone (*black dashed line*) as well as associated laryngeal structures (*black asterisk* epiglottis, *black dotted line* arytenoid) prepare to elevate from their resting position. In frames **b** and **c**, The bolus transits the pharynx then through the PES (*white asterisk*) owing to elevation of the larynx (*black arrow heads*) and propagation of the pharyngeal wave (*white arrows*). Airway protection is facilitated by laryngeal elevation, forward tilt of the arytenoid cartilages (*black dotted line*) and retroflexion of the epiglottis (*black asterisk*)

negative pressure that encourages the bolus to enter the esophagus. Lastly, PES opening depends on the relaxation and elasticity of the cricopharyngeus muscle. A more complete description of normal and abnormal PES function is found in Chaps. 5 and 10.

Vital to the pharyngeal phase of deglutition is airway protection as the bolus transits the common laryngopharyngeal compartment. The precise bolus control described above is imperative for airway protection. Additionally, a three-tiered series of protective measures occur during deglutition. The initial effect of the food bolus entering the oropharynx is vocal fold adduction, thereby closing the distal airway. Then, the supraglottis is closed by the contraction of the vestibular folds and the forward tilt of the arytenoid cartilages (Fig. 4.8b), and suprahyoid muscle contraction causes the larynx to rise approximately 1.5–2 cm. Finally, the epiglottis retroflexes as a result of laryngohyoid elevation, tongue base propulsion as well as bolus forces. This series of coordinated events prevents entry of ingested food and liquid into the airway. Inhalation is inhibited during this process, further protecting the airway from unintentional entry of food and liquid.

Suggested Reading

Aminpour S, Leonard R, Fuller SC, Belafsky PC. Pharyngeal wall differences between normal younger and older adults. Ear Nose Throat J. 2011 Apr;90(4):E1.

Nemzek WR, Katzberg RW, Van Slyke MA, Bickley LS. A reappraisal of the radiologic findings of acute inflammation of the epiglottis and supraglottic structures in adults. AJNR Am J Neuroradiol. 1995 Mar;16(3):495–502.

Leonard R, Kendall C, editors. Dysphagia assessment and treatment planning: a team approach. 3rd edn. San Diego: Plural Publishing; 2013.

Sheikh KH, Mostow SR. Epiglottitis—an increasing problem for adults. West J Med. 1989 Nov;151(5):520–524.

Chapter 5
Normal Pharyngoesophageal Segment Fluoroscopy

The upper esophageal sphincter (UES) is a 2.5–4.5 cm manometric high-pressure zone located between the pharynx and esophagus (Figs. 5.1 and 5.2). Because of its location, this region has also been referred to as the pharyngoesophageal segment (PES). The UES specifically refers to the intraluminal high-pressure zone that may be visualized on manometry. The PES refers to the anatomic components that make up the high-pressure zone. The UES and PES **are** synonymous and may be used interchangeably. The cricopharyngeus muscle (CPM) makes up only one component of the PES. The CPM is *not* synonymous with the UES and PES. The PES is modifiable with therapy and surgery. It is for this reason that a comprehensive understanding of PES fluoroscopic anatomy and physiology is essential for all swallowing clinicians (Fig. 5.3).

The PES is made up of the inferior pharyngeal constrictor (IPC), the CPM, and the most proximal cervical esophagus (Fig. 5.1). The actions of all three muscles in addition to the elastic recoil of the thyroid and cricoid cartilages against the cervical spine maintain resting tone. The function of the PES is to prevent aerophagia during respiration and phonation and to protect against aspiration of refluxed gastric and esophageal contents. The PES possesses baseline tone and remains contracted at rest. It reflexively opens during deglutition, eructation (burping), and vomiting. Distension of the esophagus, emotional stress, pharyngeal stimulation, and acid in the esophagus all reflexively tighten the PES. Of the three components that make up the PES, only the CPM contracts and relaxes during all reflex tasks.

Normal PES Opening

The act of swallowing depends upon adequate and timely PES opening. Opening of the PES depends upon muscular relaxation of the CPM, elevation of the larynx, and pharyngeal contraction. Jacob et al. (1989) described five phases of PES opening (Table 5.1). In the first phase there is an inhibition of tonic PES contraction (Fig. 5.4). This depends on muscular relaxation of the tonically active CPM. Phase I of PES opening is followed by elevation of the hyoid and larynx. Hyolaryngeal

P. C. Belafsky, M. A. Kuhn, *The Clinician's Guide to Swallowing Fluoroscopy,* DOI 10.1007/978-1-4939-1109-7_5, © Springer Science+Business Media New York 2014

Fig. 5.1 Region of the upper esophageal sphincter (UES). *IPC* inferior pharyngeal constrictor; *CPM* cricopharyngeus muscle. (Gray, Henry. Anatomy of the Human Body. Philadelphia: Lea and Febiger 1918)

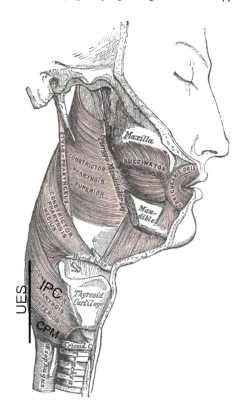

Fig. 5.2 Region of the upper esophageal sphincter (UES) on lateral fluoroscopy. *TVF* true vocal fold

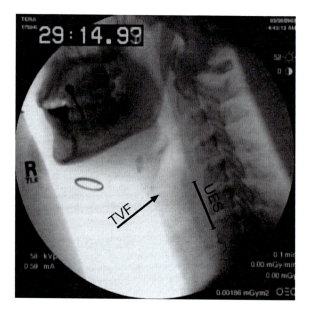

Fig. 5.3 Anatomic structures in lateral fluoroscopic view. *Yellow arrows* soft palate; *Black arrows* base of tongue; *Black dashed line* hyoid bone; *TE* tip of epiglottis; *red dotted line* aryepiglottic fold; *AC* anterior commissure; *blue dashed line* true vocal fold; *LV* laryngeal ventricle (space between true and false vocal folds); *Yellow dotted line* and *AC* arytenoid cartilage; *Black dotted line* and *CC* cricoid cartilage

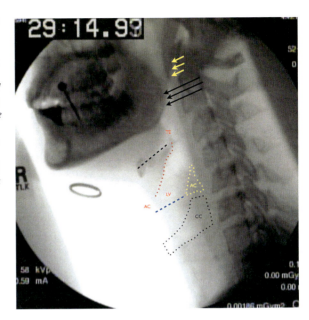

Table 5.1 Stages of PES opening

Stage	
I	Muscular relaxation of the cricopharyngeus muscle
II	Elevation of the hyoid and larynx
III	Distension of the PES through lingual and pharyngeal contraction
IV	Passive closure of the PES through elastic recoil of laryngeal cartilages
V	Active PES closure through cricopharyngeus muscle contraction

PES pharyngoesophageal segment

excursion (Phase II) provides opening of the PES (Fig. 5.5) through active distraction of the larynx and cricoid cartilages away from the cervical spine. The anterior–superior elevation also helps bring the larynx forward underneath the base of tongue and helps direct the bolus posteriorly toward the hypopharynx. The cartilages do not actually distend off of the spine to open the PES in Phase II, but the region is primed to accept the bolus in preparation for definitive opening in Phase III. The priming provided by elevation appears to be more important than muscular inhibition in Phase I. Elevation is necessary to allow a bolus to enter the PES. Muscular relaxation of the CPM without elevation will not result in PES opening. This has significant clinical implications, as swallowing in individuals with good hyolaryngeal elevation but poor CPM relaxation is possible and often encountered (CPM bar). Safe and effective swallowing in individuals who can relax their CPM but cannot elevate their larynx off of the cervical spine has not been observed. The advancing

Fig. 5.4 Phase I of UES
opening. Inhibition of tonic
UES contraction. The baseline electrical activity of the
b cricopharyngeus muscle on
EMG and *B* UES pressure
on manometry, diminishes
(*black arrow, asterisk*).
The barium bolus has been
transported to the base of the
tongue

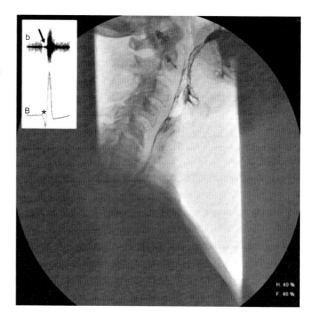

Fig. 5.5 Phase II of UES
opening. The larynx (L) and
hyoid (H) are elevated, priming the UES for acceptance
of the bolus and distension in
Phase III. The thyroid cartilage remains apposed to the
cervical spine and the UES
remains closed (*black line*)

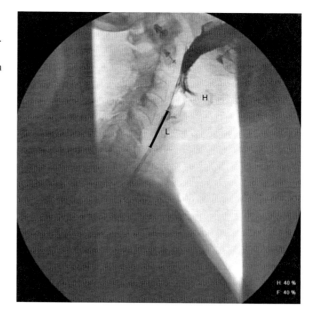

bolus will reach a closed PES and follow the path of least resistance into the airway.
The third phase of PES opening involves distension of the PES through bolus size
and weight (Fig. 5.6). This phase relies upon pharyngeal and lingual peristalsis to
propel the bolus past the spacious hypopharynx, through the closed but primed PES,

Fig. 5.6 Phase III of UES opening. Distension of the UES by bolus size and weight. This requires adequate lingual and pharyngeal pressure to distract the thyroid cartilage (*TC*) off of the cervical spine (*CS*). The UES opens only as little as required to accommodate the advancing bolus (*asterisk*). *CP* cricopharyngeus muscle

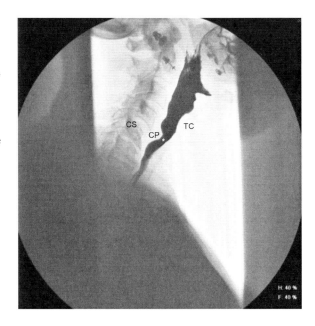

behind the elevating hyolaryngeal complex, and into the cervical esophagus. The elasticity of the elevating PES allows it to be opened by the increasing pressure exerted by the passing bolus. If there is inadequate lingual and pharyngeal contraction, the bolus will not exert enough pressure and the PES will not open. The bolus will again follow the path of least resistance and threaten the airway. The PES cannot adequately be evaluated if lingual and pharyngeal contractility are ineffectual. This is a major limitation of the VFSS, as PES pathology (e.g., CPM bar, stricture, web) cannot be assessed in persons with a significantly weakened tongue or pharynx. In Phase IV of PES opening, the elasticity of the PES causes passive collapse and closure as the bolus passes (Fig. 5.7). The final phase of PES opening, Phase V, involves PES closure through active contraction of the CPM (Fig. 5.8). A disease process that affects any one of the five phases of PES opening can cause the symptom of dysphagia and objective evidence of swallowing dysfunction.

The VFSS is the current gold standard diagnostic test for the evaluation of the PES. The distended PES is challenging to visualize because of the rapid transit of contrast, its short length, and its tonic sphincteric closure. The cartilaginous framework of the larynx directly apposes the cervical spine and flexible endoscopy is insufficient in evaluating this region. The cartilage must be distended off of the spine in order to adequately evaluate the back of the cricoid cartilage and esophageal inlet. This is only possible when the area is distended with a laryngoscope or dilator (Fig. 5.9). Stop-motion fluoroscopic imaging at a capture rate of 30 frames per second (fps) is the only available method of precisely evaluating the essential components of PES function (laryngohyoid elevation, pharyngeal contractility, PES

Fig. 5.7 Phase IV of UES
opening. The bolus has
passed into the esophagus
and the elastic recoil of the
descending thyroid cartilage
(*TC*) toward the cervical
spine (*CS*) causes passive
closure of the UES (*black
line*)

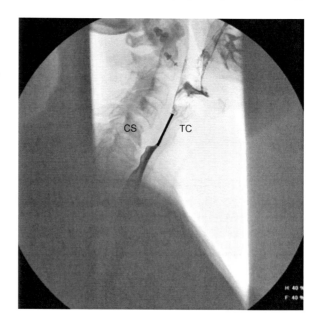

Fig. 5.8 Phase V of UES
opening. The hyoid bone
(*H*) and thyroid cartilage
(*TC*) have descended to their
pre-swallow positions and
the PES closes through active
contraction of the cricopharyngeus (*CP*) muscle. There
is post swallow increased
electrical activity of the CP
muscle on electromyography
(*short arrow*) and a transient
elevation of UES manometric
pressure above baseline on
manometry (*long arrow*)

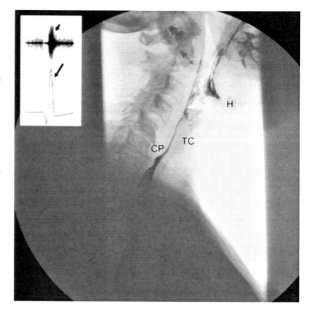

opening, and pharyngeal-PES coordination). Capture rates less than 30 fps are inadequate to comprehensively evaluate this region.

Normal PES opening increases with enlarging bolus size and decreases with
advancing age. The PES will enlarge only as much as necessary to accommodate
the ingested material. Maximum PES opening in normal individuals <65 years of

Fig. 5.9 Endoscopic view
of the upper esophageal
sphincter. The larynx is
distended anteriorly off
of the cervical spine by a
radial expansion balloon
dilator (*BD*) in a patient
with a pharyngoesophageal
web (*arrowheads*). *CPM*
cricopharyngeus muscle;
PS right pyriform sinus; *AC*
back of arytenoid cartilage;
long arrow posterior cricoid
region; *short arrow* laryngeal
surface of epiglottis

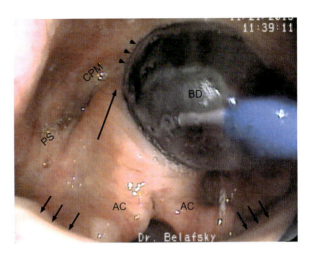

Fig. 5.10 Lateral fluoroscopic view of a non-
obstructing cricopharyngeus
muscle bar (*asterisk*). UES
opening (*white line*) is within
normal limits (>0.60 cm)

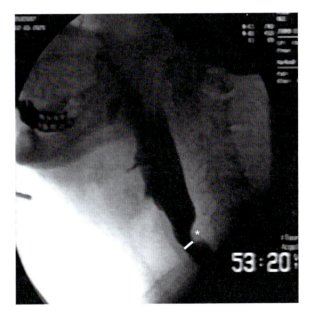

age ranges from 0.39 cm with a 1 cc bolus to 0.90 cm with a 20 cc bolus. The lower
limit of normal (mean less 1 SD) is 0.6 cm. A CPM bar is considered obstructing
when the maximum PES opening is <0.60 cm. We frequently encounter individuals
with a CPM bar who have normal PES opening (Fig. 5.10). In fact, 30% of elderly
nondysphagic persons have evidence of a CPM bar on fluoroscopy. The presence of
a CPM bar does *not* imply the existence of dysphagia or objective evidence of swallowing dysfunction. A comprehensive discussion of abnormal PES fluoroscopic
findings is presented in Chap. 10.

An assessment of laryngohyoid elevation (Phase II of PES opening) is essential in the evaluation of PES dynamics. An individual who cannot adequately elevate the larynx off of the spine will not be able to open the PES, even after CP myotomy. Normal elevation varies by age, gender, and bolus size. Normal hyolaryngeal elevation ranges from 2.49 cm with a 1 cc bolus in women < 65 years of age to 4.06 cm with a 20 cc bolus in men > 65 years of age. Performing CPM surgery on an individual with poor laryngeal elevation is hazardous and likely to fail. In these cases a laryngohyoid suspension procedure may be added to the surgical myotomy.

An assessment of pharyngeal strength (phase III of PES opening) is also essential in the evaluation of PES dynamics. A pharynx that cannot generate adequate intra-bolus pressure to distend the elevated larynx off of the spine cannot adequately open the PES. The VFSS can provide an objective measure of pharyngeal contractility. The pharyngeal constriction ratio (PCR) is a validated surrogate measure of pharyngeal strength on fluoroscopy and is further described in Chap. 7. The PCR is the maximal pharyngeal area during passage of a bolus divided by the pharyngeal area with the bolus held in the mouth. A normal PCR approaches zero. As pharyngeal constriction diminishes, the PCR increases. Individuals with a PCR greater than 0.25 are three times more likely to aspirate (95% CI = 1.7, 5.1). Individuals with a weak pharynx and an elevated PCR have a more guarded prognosis for surgery aimed at improving PES opening such as CPM myotomy, laryngohyoid elevation, or PES dilation.

An evaluation of the posterior cricoid (PC) region on fluoroscopy is essential in the assessment of PES function. Fluoroscopic evaluation of this area is a challenge and requires the administration of a large bolus of barium to adequately distend the region. The PES cannot be accurately assessed if an individual cannot safely consume a large bolus of contrast (10–20 ml). We differentiate anatomy in this region as being a PC finding or a posterior hypopharyngeal finding. The PC region is defined as the area immediately adjacent to the posterior rim of the cricoid cartilage on the anterior wall of the esophageal inlet. The posterior hypopharyngeal region is defined as the area on the posterior hypopharyngeal wall at the most cranial region of the esophageal inlet (Fig. 5.11). Posterior hypopharyngeal findings include CPM bars and diverticuli (Zenker). A nonobstructing CPM bar (PES opening > 0.6 cm) is considered normal (Fig. 5.10). A detailed description of posterior hypopharyngeal pathology is presented in Chap. 10.

PC findings include an unremarkable PC region, a PC arch impression, a PC plication, and a cricopharyngeal web. Only webs are considered pathologic. An analysis of several hundred VFSS revealed PC findings in over 50%. The most common finding was a PC plication, seen in 23% of healthy volunteers and in 30% of dysphagic individuals ($p > 0.05$). The PC plication is defined as a fluoroscopic protrusion into the barium stream on the posterior surface of the cricoid arch that rises with the swallow (Fig. 5.12). It is considered a normal variant. We hypothesize that the PC plication represents a fold of mucosa overlying slips of muscle that arise from the longitudinal layer of the esophagus and extend up to the midline ridge of the PC arch. A large barium bolus maximally distends the UES and can delineate

Fig. 5.11 Posterior cricoid (*black arrows*) and posterior hypopharyngeal (*white arrowheads*) regions on lateral fluoroscopic view

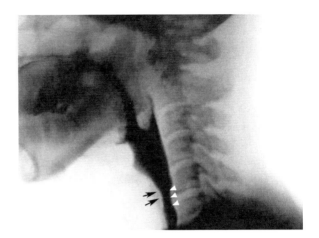

Fig. 5.12 Posterior cricoid plication (*black arrow*)

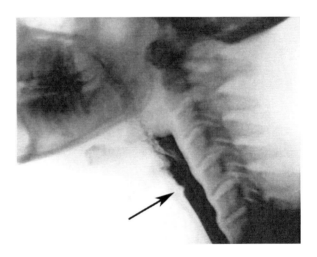

these mucosa-covered fibers. The second most common PC region finding is a PC arch impression, seen in 16 % of healthy volunteers and in 16 % of dysphagic individuals ($p > 0.05$; Fig. 5.13). The PC arch impression is a fluoroscopic outline of the posterior arch of the cricoid cartilage that elevates with the swallow. It is considered a normal variant. The third most common PC finding is a web. Pharyngoesophageal or cricopharyngeal webs are seen in 7 % of healthy volunteers and in 14 % of dysphagic individuals ($p < 0.05$). They are considered pathologic. CP webs are located on the anterior wall of the esophageal inlet caudal to the cricoid arch. Webs are thin, do not change in shape, and are typically located at the level of the fifth cervical vertebrae. The indentation of the web on the posterior arch of the cricoid corresponds to a similar indentation on the adjacent posterior hypopharyngeal wall (Fig. 5.14). CP webs are discussed in detail in Chap. 10.

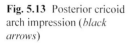

Fig. 5.13 Posterior cricoid arch impression (*black arrows*)

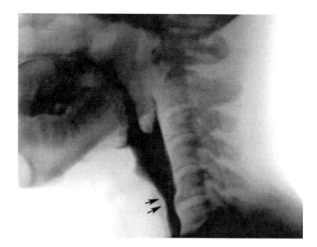

Fig. 5.14 Cricopharyngeal web (*black arrows*)

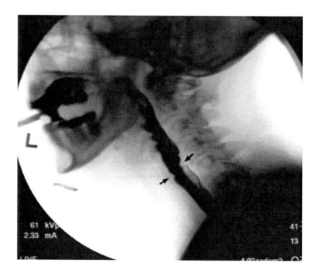

Airway Protection

The laryngopharynx is the common cavity responsible for the vital roles of breathing and swallowing. Airway protection during deglutition is the most important phylogenetic function of the region. Airway protection relies on a three-tiered layer of defense. The first tier involves laryngeal elevation and epiglottic inversion. The combined effect of laryngohyoid elevation and lingual contraction inverts the epiglottis and closes the airway by elevating the arytenoid cartilages against the petiole of the epiglottis. This action also directs the bolus away from the airway toward the primed PES posteriorly. The second and third tiers of airway protection involve closure of the false and true vocal cords (Figs. 5.15 and 5.16). A process that alters any one of the layers of airway protection can result in laryngeal penetration or aspiration.

Fig. 5.15 Lateral fluoroscopic view before the initiation of airway protection. The larynx is in its resting position and the pharyngoesophageal segment is closed (*yellow line*). The tip of the epiglottis has not yet inverted (*dotted red line*) and the arytenoid cartilage (*dotted blue line*) has not yet elevated against the petiole of the epiglottis (*P*). The vocal fold has not adducted (*dotted black line*) and the airway is open (*asterisk*)

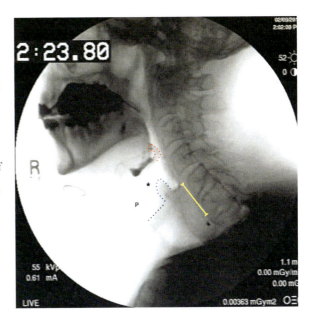

Fig. 5.16 Lateral fluoroscopic view during airway protection. The tip of the epiglottis has inverted (*dotted red line*) and the bolus is diverted posteriorly into the expanding pharyngoesophageal segment (*yellow line*). The arytenoid cartilage (*dotted blue line*) has elevated against the petiole of the epiglottis and the airway is closed (*asterisk*). Closure of the false and true vocal folds (*dotted black line*) provides additional protection

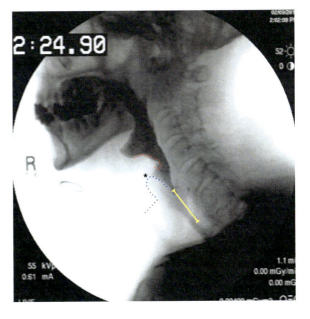

The unique ability of fluoroscopy to objectively evaluate the interrelationship between airway protection, laryngohyoid elevation, lingual and pharyngeal contractility, and PES opening makes the VFSS an essential aspect of the comprehensive dysphagia workup.

Suggested Reading

Allen JE, White CJ, Leonard RJ, Belafsky PC. Prevalence of penetration and aspiration on videofluoroscopy in normal individuals without dysphagia. Otolaryngol Head Neck Surg. 2010 Feb;142(2):208–13.

Allen JE, White CJ, Leonard RJ, Belafsky PC. Posterior cricoid region fluoroscopic findings: the posterior cricoid plication. Dysphagia. 2011 Sep;26(3):272–6.

Aminpour S, Leonard R, Fuller SC, Belafsky PC. Pharyngeal wall differences between normal younger and older adults. Ear Nose Throat J. 2011 April;90(4):E1.

Belafsky PC. Manual control of the upper esophageal sphincter. Laryngoscope. 2010 April;120 Suppl 1:S1–S16.

Jacob P, Kahrilas PJ, Logemann JA, Shah V, Ha T. Upper esophageal sphincter opening and modulation during swallowing. Gastroenterology. 1989 Dec;97(6):1469–78.

Kendall KA, Leonard RJ, McKenzie SW. Accommodation to changes in bolus viscosity in normal deglutition: a videofluoroscopic study. Ann Otol Rhinol Laryngol. 2001 Nov;110(11):1059–65.

Kendall KA, Leonard RJ, McKenzie S. Airway protection: evaluation with videofluoroscopy. Dysphagia. 2004 Spring;19(2):65–70.

Leonard R, Kendall C, editors. Dysphagia assessment and treatment planning: a team approach. 2nd edn. San Diego: Plural Publishing; 2007.

Leonard RJ, Kendall KA, McKenzie S, Gonçalves MI, Walker A. Structural displacements in normal swallowing: a videofluoroscopic study. Dysphagia. 2000 Summer;15(3):146–52.

Leonard R, Kendall KA, McKenzie S. Structural displacements affecting pharyngeal constriction in nondysphagic elderly and nonelderly adults. Dysphagia. 2004 Spring;19(2):133–41.

Leonard R, Kendall K, McKenzie S. UES opening and cricopharyngeal bar in nondysphagic elderly and nonelderly adults. Dysphagia. 2004 Summer;19(3):182–91.

Leonard R, Belafsky PC, Rees CJ. Relationship between fluoroscopic and manometric measures of pharyngeal constriction: the pharyngeal constriction ratio. Ann Otol Rhinol Laryngol. 2006 Dec;115(12):897–901.

Leonard R, Rees CJ, Belafsky P, Allen J. Fluoroscopic surrogate for pharyngeal strength: the pharyngeal constriction ratio (PCR). Dysphagia. 2011 Mar;26(1):13–7.

Shaker R, Belafsky PC, Postma GN, Easterling C, editors. Principles of deglutition: a multidisciplinary text for swallowing and its disorders. New York: Springer; 2012.

Shaker R, Belafsky PC, Postma GN, Easterling C, editors. Manual of diagnostic and therapeutic techniques for disorders of deglutition. New York: Springer; 2012.

Chapter 6
Normal Esophageal Fluoroscopy

The esophagus is an approximately 25 cm-long organ that connects the hypopharynx to the gastric cardia. There are four compressions that are visualized on normal esophageal fluoroscopy. The first compression is that of the pharyngoesophageal segment (PES) (Chap. 5; Fig. 6.1). This region connects the hypopharynx to the cervical esophagus and is identified at approximately 17 cm from the oral commissure or nasal vestibule on esophagoscopy. The second compression is visualized endoscopicaly at 24 cm from the oral commissure and is caused by the arch of the aorta (Figs. 6.2, 6.3, and 6.4). Crossing posteriorly to the left main stem bronchus at 28 cm causes a third indentation significantly less prominent than the aorta. The final compression is caused by the pinch of the diaphragmatic hiatus at approximately 40 cm from the oral commissure (Figs. 6.5 and 6.6).

As the PES closes, esophageal peristalsis transports an advancing bolus along the entire esophageal body through a relaxed lower esophageal sphincter (LES). The LES relaxes with the initiation of the pharyngeal swallow and remains open until the bolus advances into the stomach. Although the LES relaxes with the initiation of the pharyngeal swallow on manometry, the LES does not open on fluoroscopy until it is distended by an advancing bolus. The normal swallow-induced esophageal contraction is referred to as *primary peristalsis*. Peristalsis is visualized fluoroscopically as a stripping wave (Fig. 6.7). A normal esophageal stripping wave transmits a bolus at approximately 2 cm/s. Thus, a bolus should clear the normal 25 cm esophagus in less than 15 s. Liquid barium should proceed throughout its entire length in one smooth motion. Barium tablets may proceed more rapidly in an upright individual as transit may bypass peristalsis and the tablet may drop into the stomach by gravity alone. The esophagus may shorten up to 3 cm during bolus transit in response to the normal contraction of the longitudinal esophageal muscle. *Secondary peristalsis* occurs irrespective of a pharyngeal swallow. It occurs in response to esophageal chemical (acid) or mechanical (distension) stimulation. The secondary contractile stripping wave occurs similar to the primary wave but initiates at the level of the stimulation and not in the pharynx. Secondary peristalsis is considered a function of normal esophageal biomechanics. It is an essential mechanism to clear the esophagus of retained and regurgitated food (reflux). *Tertiary peristalsis* is simultaneous, isolated, nonperistaltic esophageal contractions that occur

P. C. Belafsky, M. A. Kuhn, *The Clinician's Guide to Swallowing Fluoroscopy,*
DOI 10.1007/978-1-4939-1109-7_6, © Springer Science+Business Media New York 2014

Fig. 6.1 Esophageal
compression on anterior–
posterior videofluoroscopic
esophagram caused by upper
esophageal sphincter (*black
arrows*)

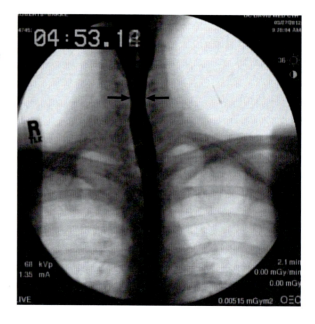

Fig. 6.2 Diagram of thoracic
compressions on the esophagus caused by the aorta and
left mainstem bronchus.
(Anatomy of the Esophagus.
Authors: Najam, Azmeena,
Ajani, Jaffer, Markman,
Maurie, Book title: Atlas
of Cancer, Published Date:
2003-01-16)

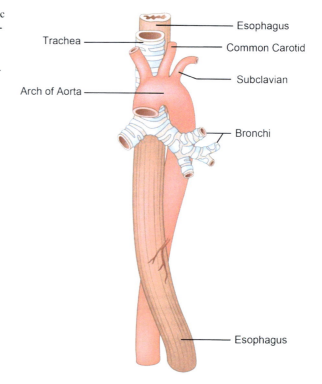

Fig. 6.3 Esophageal
compressions on anterior-
posterior videofluoroscopic
esophagram caused by upper
esophageal sphincter (*short
black arrows*), aortic arch
(*black arrowheads*), and left
mainstem bronchus (*long
black arrow*)

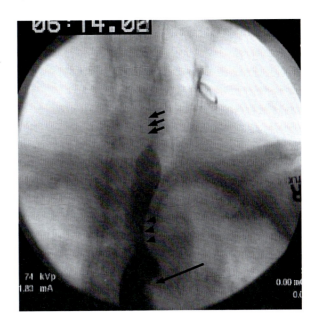

Fig. 6.4 Esophageal compressions on esophagoscopy
caused by aortic arch (*black
arrows*) and left mainstem
bronchus (*asterisk*)

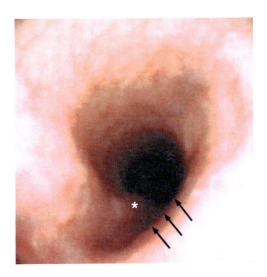

irrespective of coordinated peristalsis (Fig. 6.8). They are nonpropulsive and are
considered a sign of esophageal dysmotility. They are not part of normal esophageal
function. Profound tertiary contractions can be seen in esophageal spasm and give
the appearance of a corkscrew esophagus (Chap. 11). They may be associated with
underlying gastroesophageal reflux.

The region of the proximal third of the esophagus on fluoroscopy above the aortic compression is referred to as the esophageal dead zone. This area corresponds to

Fig. 6.5 Esophageal compression on videofluoroscopic esophagram caused by the diaphragmatic pinch (*black arrows*)

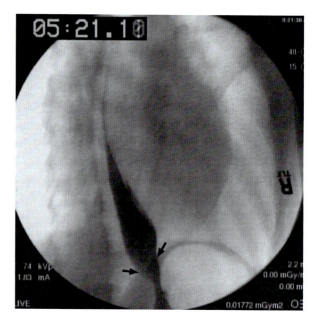

Fig. 6.6 Esophageal compression on esophagoscopy caused by the diaphragmatic pinch (*black arrows*). Gastric rugae (*black arrowheads*) extend above the diaphragm indicating the presence of a hiatal hernia

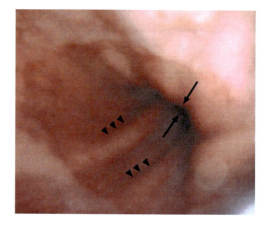

the manometric low-pressure zone that normally occurs at the junction of esophageal striated and smooth muscle (Fig. 6.9). Barium liquid or tablet stasis in this region is frequently encountered and small transit delays in the dead zone may be considered a variant of normal.

The distal "tubular" esophagus flares out above the esophagogastric junction (EGJ) to form the esophageal vestibule (Fig. 6.10). The tubulo-vestibular junction occurs approximately 2 cm above the EGJ and the apex of the vestibule is a landmark often utilized to identify the location of the EGJ (Fig. 6.10).

The LES is an approximately 4 cm high-pressure zone located between the esophagus and gastric cardia. The diaphragmatic hiatus provides the primary pres-

Fig. 6.7 Esophageal stripping wave (*black arrow-
heads*) propelling the barium
bolus through the distal
esophagus into the stomach

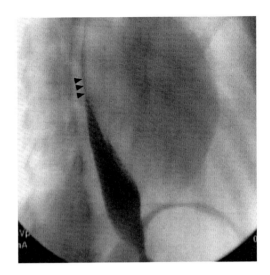

Fig. 6.8 Tertiary contractions
(*black arrows*) on fluoroscopic esophagram

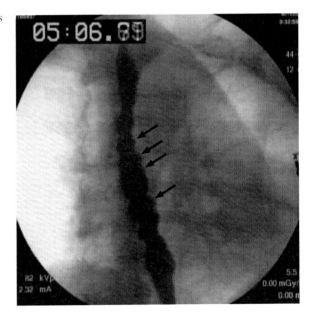

sure contribution to this region and is an essential fluoroscopic landmark. The hypertrophied smooth muscle of the LES contributes secondary tone. The proximal-
most aspect of the intrinsic smooth muscle of the LES is seen fluoroscopically as
the esophageal A-ring (Fig. 6.11). A-rings represent normal fluoroscopic anatomy.
Severely enlarged A-rings may be a rare cause of pathologic obstruction (Chap. 11).
The esophagus in the region of the LES is attached to the diaphragm by the phreno-
esophageal ligament (PEL). The attachment of the LES to the crura by the PEL

Fig. 6.9 Region of esophageal dead zone (*double-headed black arrow*). A 13 mm barium tablet (*asterisk*) is stuck above the aortic compression (*A*). This region corresponds to a region of low contraction pressure at the junction of esophageal striated and smooth muscle. It is a frequent site of esophageal stasis

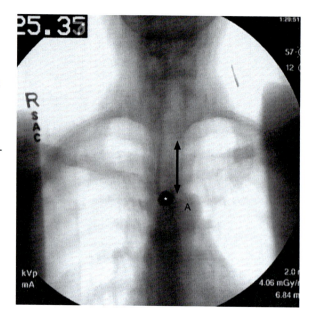

Fig. 6.10 Videofluoroscopic esophageal image displaying the junction of the tubular esophagus (*yellow lines*) and the esophageal vestibule (*blue lines*). The tubulo-vestibular junction (*black arrow*) is approximately 2 cm above the esophagogastric junction (*white dotted line*) at the apex of the esophageal vestibule

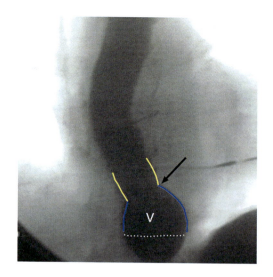

causes the LES to move with respiration. Weakening of the PEL is a cause of hiatal hernia, and the separation of the intrinsic smooth muscle LES from the barrier effect of the diaphragmatic pinch as occurs with hernia development is a major contribution to reflux disease (Chap. 11).

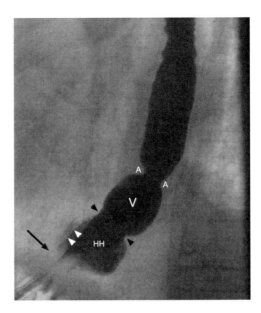

Fig. 6.11 Videofluoroscopic anatomy of the distal esophagus in the right anterior oblique view. The region of the lower esophageal sphincter (LES) is a 3–4 cm region of elevated pressure in the distal esophagus. Both the intrinsic smooth muscle component of the LES and the pressure provided by the diaphragm contribute to pressure at the LES. The most proximal aspect of the intrinsic smooth muscle component can be seen as a compression at the tubulo-vestibular junction (*A*). In this image, the gastric rugae (*white arrowheads*) have migrated above the diaphragm (*black arrow*) indicating the presence of a hiatal hernia (*HH*). Compression from a Schatzki's B-ring (*black arrowheads*) can also be seen at the distal aspect of the esophageal vestibule (*V*) at the esophagogastric junction

Suggested Reading

Levine MS, Rubesin SE. Diseases of the esophagus: diagnosis with esophagography. Radiology. 2005 Nov;237(2):414–27.

Shaker R, Belafsky PC, Postma GN, Easterling C, editors. Principles of deglutition: a multidisciplinary text for swallowing and its disorders. New York: Springer; 2012.

Shaker R, Belafsky PC, Postma GN, Easterling C, editors. Manual of diagnostic and therapeutic techniques for disorders of deglutition. New York: Springer; 2012.

Chapter 7
Objective Measures on Videofluo⁷ Swallow Studies

Subjective assessment by experienced clinicians is unable to accurately determine parameters of the videofluoroscopic swallow study (VFSS). Values such as pharyngoesophageal segment (PES) opening, laryngeal elevation, pharyngeal area, and transit times cannot be reliably determined without measuring. Intra- and inter-rater agreement by experienced clinicians for the subjective assessment of some VFSS variables is as low as 70 %. The calculation of objective measures is essential to differentiate normal from disordered swallowing, to monitor the effects of time and intervention, and to provide precise outcome variables for research. At our center, we have integrated the objective measures of timing, displacement, and area as described and refined by Leonard and McKenzie since the 1990s.

Objective VFSS data have been collected on large populations of young (less than 65 years) and elderly (65 years or greater) men and women without swallowing disorders. These data are essential to establish normal values and to compare specific patient populations with age and gender matched controls (Table 7.1).

In order to accurately determine objective measures from fluoroscopic examinations, the studies must be acquired with uniform body positioning, barium density, distance to the imaging source, consistent resolution and capture rates, and the use of quality recording and reviewing equipment. Performing each study according to a standardized protocol is essential to ensure a high degree of precision and reproducibility (Chap. 2). Most measures are made from the sequence when the largest bolus (usually 20 cc) is swallowed. Although normative data are available for smaller bolus sizes, these measurements have less clinical utility than assessment with larger volumes. Acquiring timing measures requires a counter that displays time to the hundredth second superimposed on the fluoroscopic recording; we use the Horita Video Stopwatch VS-50 (Horita, Mission Vijeo, CA) (Fig. 7.1). If this equipment is not available, timing measures may be calculated by hand when frame number and rates are known. Most measures are obtained in the lateral fluoroscopic view and require two frames for comparison. The first frame is the "hold" or "pseudo-rest" position, which is obtained while the subject holds a 1 cc bolus in the mouth (Fig. 7.1a). Holding the 1 cc bolus in the oral cavity provides a standardized anatomic position for reproducible assessment. The comparison image is the frame at maximum displacement of the structure of interest (hyoid, larynx, pharynx).

7.1 Normative mean values of timing, displacement, and area for males and females with c bolus

easure	Value (20 cc bolus)	
	Age < 65 years	Age ≥ 65 years
Oropharyngeal transit time (s)	0.23	0.42
Hypopharyngeal transit time (s)	0.64	0.77
Airway closure duration (s)	0.72	0.85
PES opening duration (s)	0.50	0.64
Laryngeal elevation (cm)	1.25 (male), 1.07 (female)	1.58 (male), 1.23 (female)
PES opening (lateral, cm)	0.90	0.80
PES opening (anterior–posterior, cm)	1.69 (male), 1.35 (female)	1.54 (male), 1.40 (female)
Pharyngeal area (hold, cm²)	7.2 (male), 6.5 (female)	11.4 (male), 8.1 (female)
Pharyngeal constriction ratio	0.06 (male), 0.03 (female)	0.28 (male), 0.14 (female)

PES pharyngoesophageal segment

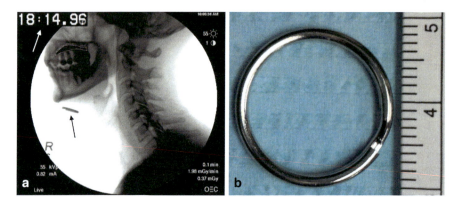

Fig. 7.1 Lateral fluoroscopic view representing the "hold" or reference position, obtained while the subject holds a 1-cc bolus in the mouth (*white dotted line*). Also shown is a counter measuring time to one-hundredth of a second (*white arrow*) and a ring 1.9 cm in diameter (*black arrow*). Same ring placed for calibration

Obtaining displacement measures requires the use of digital measuring software; at our center, we use Universal Desktop Ruler for distance determination (http://www. avp.soft) and ImageJ for area calculation (http://rsbweb.nih.gov/ij). Pixels that are digitally measured using these programs are converted to centimeters through calibration. In order to calibrate the onscreen tools, a ring of known diameter is placed on the chin (lateral view, Fig. 7.1a) or neck (anterior–posterior view) for reference. A keychain, washer, or coin may be used for this purpose (Fig. 7.1b).

The objective assessment of the VFSS is broadly classified into measurements of timing, displacement, and area (Table 7.2). Timing measures (in seconds) are further subclassified into bolus transit times and timing of anatomic structure movement.

Table 7.2 Measures of timing, displacement, and area

Measure	Definition
Timing (s)	
Oropharyngeal transit time	Time from when bolus head first passes posterior nasal spine to time bolus head enters base of vallecula (Fig. 7.2)
Hypopharyngeal transit time	Time from when bolus head exits the vallecula to time when bolus tale exits PES (Fig. 7.3)
Total pharyngeal transit time	The addition of oropharyngeal and hypopharyngeal transit times
Airway closure duration	Time from when arytenoid cartilage approximates petiole of epiglottis to when epiglottis returns to its preswallow resting position (Fig. 7.4)
PES opening duration	Time from when PES first opens for bolus entry to when it first closes behind the bolus (Fig. 7.5)
Displacement (cm)	
Maximum laryngeal elevation	Difference of the distance between the hyoid and larynx at rest and at maximum approximation (Fig. 7.6)
PES opening (lateral)	Distance at the narrowest point of opening between C3 and C6 on lateral fluoroscopic view (Fig. 7.7)
PES opening (anterior–posterior)	Distance at the narrowest point of opening between the pharynx and esophagus on anterior–posterior view (Fig. 7.8)
Area (cm²)	
Maximum pharyngeal area	Pharyngeal area in hold position (Fig. 7.9a)
Pharyngeal constriction ratio	Ratio of pharyngeal area at maximal constriction (Fig. 7.9b) to pharyngeal area at hold (Fig. 7.9a)

PES pharyngoesophageal segment

Timing Measures

Bolus Transit Times

The initiation of bolus transit time or "time zero" begins when the head of the bolus passes the posterior nasal spine (Fig. 7.2a). This is the reference point for other bolus transit measures. Oropharyngeal transit time is measured from the time the head of the bolus passes the posterior nasal spine until it enters the base of the vallecula (Fig. 7.2b). Hypopharyngeal transit time is measured from the time the head of the bolus leaves the base of the vallecula (Fig. 7.3a) until the time the tail of the bolus exits the PES (Fig. 7.3b). Total pharyngeal transit time is the simple addition of both times. Normative data for these timing measures are in Table 7.1. Prolonged pharyngeal transit times increase the duration that a bolus may threaten the airway and are associated with a significantly increased risk of aspiration pneumonia.

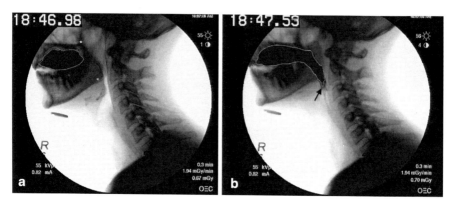

Fig. 7.2 Lateral fluoroscopic views for determining oropharynageal transit time. (**a**) The time when the head of the bolus (white dotted line) first passes the posterior nasal spine (*white asterisk*) is subtracted from (**b**) the time when the head of the bolus (*white dotted line*) enters and exits the base of the vallecula (*black arrow*)

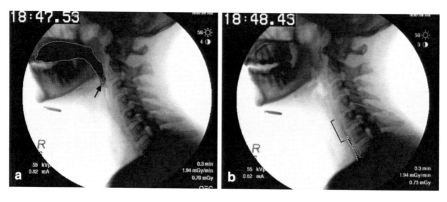

Fig. 7.3 Lateral fluoroscopic views for determining hypopharyngeal transit time. (**a**) The time when the head of the bolus (*white dotted line*) leaves the base of the vallecula (*black arrow*) is subtracted from (**b**) the time the tail of the bolus (*white dotted line*) leaves the PES (*black bracket*)

Anatomic Structure Movement Times

The most clinically relevant timing measures of anatomic structure movement are airway closure duration and PES opening duration. Airway closure duration is measured from the time the arytenoid cartilage approximates the petiole of the epiglottis (Fig. 7.4a) until the time the epiglottis resumes its preswallow resting position (Fig. 7.4b). PES opening duration is measured from the time the head of the bolus enters the PES until the time the PES closes on the bolus (Fig. 7.5). Reduced airway closure duration increases aspiration risk and provides a useful target for swallowing therapy. Shortened PES opening duration may also increase aspiration risk and be targeted with therapy.

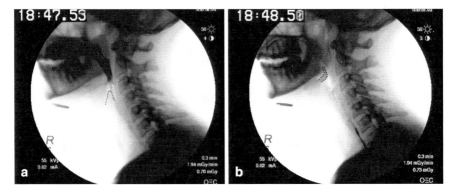

Fig. 7.4 Lateral fluoroscopic views used to determine airway closure duration. (**a**) The time at which the arytenoid (*black dotted line*) makes contact with the petiole of the epiglottis is subtracted from (**b**) the time when the epiglottis (*black dotted line*) returns to its preswallow position

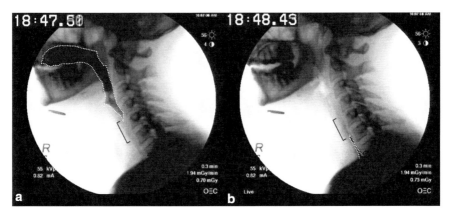

Fig. 7.5 Lateral fluoroscopic views for measuring PES opening duration. (**a**) The time when the head of the bolus (*white dotted line*) first enters the PES (*black bracket*) is subtracted from (**b**) the time when the tail of the bolus (*dotted line*) leaves the PES (*black bracket*)

Displacement Measures

These measures include laryngeal elevation and PES opening. Objective measures of hyoid elevation exist but are more tedious to acquire. In addition, elevation of the hyoid is a surrogate measure of laryngeal elevation and has less clinical utility (Chap. 5—Phase II of PES opening). Acquisition begins with establishing a reference frame that is referred to as the "hold" position and is captured while a 1 cc bolus is held in the oral cavity (Fig. 7.1a). Laryngeal elevation is measured by comparing the distance between the hyoid and larynx at rest or hold position (Fig. 7.6a) and at maximum approximation (Fig. 7.6b). Diminished laryngeal elevation can be targeted with both therapy and surgery. PES opening on fluoroscopy is

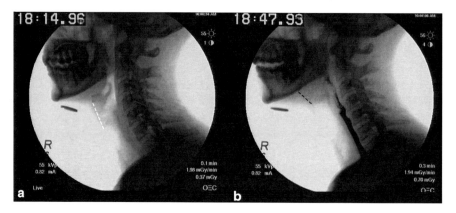

Fig. 7.6 Lateral fluoroscopic views used to calculate maximum laryngeal elevation. The distance between the hyoid and larynx at hold position (*white dashed line*) is compared to the distance at maximum approximation (*black dashed line*)

Fig. 7.7 Lateral fluoro-scopic view demonstrating maximum PES opening (*white line*), measured at narrowest point between C3 and C6. Also seen is a posterior cricoid impression (*black asterisk*)

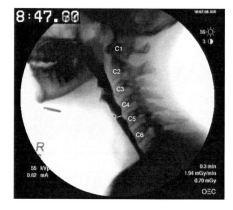

simply defined as the narrowest point of opening between C3 and C6 in the lateral fluoroscopic view (Fig. 7.7) and the narrowest point of opening between the pharynx and esophagus on the anterior–posterior view (Fig. 7.8). Impaired PES opening can be caused by poor cricopharyngeus muscle relaxation, diminished laryngeal elevation and pharyngeal contraction, web, and stenosis (Chap. 10). These findings may be targeted with both therapy and surgery.

Area Measurement

The pharyngeal area at rest is calculated by outlining the limits of the pharynx with onscreen tools provided by ImageJ (http://rsbweb.nih.gov/ij). The area is determined by a line drawn from the posterior nasal spine to the posterior pharyngeal

Fig. 7.8 Anterior–posterior fluoroscopic view demonstrating PES opening (*white line*), the distance at the narrowest point of opening between the pharynx (*P*) and esophagus (*E*)

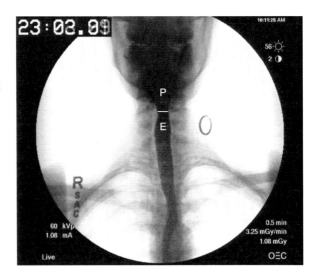

wall at the level of the tubercle of the atlas to a line drawn from arytenoid to the epiglottis (Fig. 7.9a). The program will determine the area of the outlined space automatically (cm^2). Normative values for pharyngeal area at rest are presented in Table 7.1. An enlarged pharyngeal area is associated with a weak pharynx and poor constriction and is a risk factor for aspiration. A more accurate surrogate measure of pharyngeal strength is the pharyngeal constriction ratio (PCR).

The PCR is a surrogate measure of pharyngeal clearance pressure, traditionally measured by pharyngeal manometry. It is calculated by dividing the lateral pharyngeal area during maximal contraction (Fig. 7.9b) by the area with a 1 cc bolus held in the oral cavity (Fig. 7.9a). A normal PCR approaches zero. As PCR increases, pharyngeal contractility diminishes. Individuals with a PCR greater than 0.25 are three times more likely to aspirate.

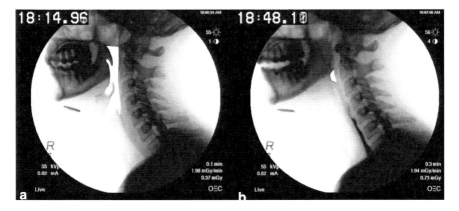

Fig. 7.9 Lateral fluoroscopic view showing (**a**) PAhold, the pharyngeal area in the "hold" position (*white shading*) and (**b**) PAmax, the pharyngeal area during maximum pharyngeal constriction

Suggested Reading

Allen J, White CJ, Leonard R, Belafsky PC. Effect of cricopharyngeus muscle surgery on the pharynx. Laryngoscope. 2010 Aug;120(8):1498–1503.

Belafsky PC, Rees CJ, Allen J, Leonard RJ. Pharyngeal dilation in cricopharyngeus muscle dysfunction and Zenker diverticulum. Laryngoscope. 2010 May;120(5):889–94.

Johnson ER, McKenzie SW. Kinematic pharyngeal transit times in myopathy: evaluation for dysphagia. Dysphagia. 1993;8(1):35–40.

Johnson ER, McKenzie SW, Rosenquist CJ, Lieberman JS, Sievers AE. Dysphagia following stroke: quantitative evaluation of pharyngeal transit times. Archives Phys Med Rehabil. 1992 May;73(5):419–23.

Kendall KA, McKenzie S, Leonard RJ, Goncalves MI, Walker A. Timing of events in normal swallowing: a videofluoroscopic study. Dysphagia. 2000 Spring;15(2):74–83.

Leonard R, Kendall C, editors. Dysphagia assessment and treatment planning: a team approach. 2nd edn. San Diego: Plural Publishing; 2007.

Leonard R, Belafsky P. Dysphagia following cervical spine surgery with anterior instrumentation: evidence from fluoroscopic swallow studies. Spine. 2011 Dec;36(25):2217–23.

Leonard RJ, Kendall KA, McKenzie S, Goncalves MI, Walker A. Structural displacements in normal swallowing: a videofluoroscopic study. Dysphagia. 2000 Summer;15(3):146–52.

Leonard RJ, Kendall KA, Johnson R, McKenzie S. Swallowing in myotonic muscular dystrophy: a videofluoroscopic study. Arch Phys Med Rehabil. 2001 July;82(7):979–85.

Leonard R, Kendall K, McKenzie S. UES opening and cricopharyngeal bar in nondysphagic elderly and nonelderly adults. Dysphagia. 2004 Summer;19(3):182–91.

Leonard R, Kendall KA, McKenzie S. Structural displacements affecting pharyngeal constriction in nondysphagic elderly and nonelderly adults. Dysphagia. 2004 Spring;19(2):133–41.

Leonard R, Belafsky PC, Rees CJ. Relationship between fluoroscopic and manometric measures of pharyngeal constriction: the pharyngeal constriction ratio. Ann Otol Rhinol Laryngol. 2006 Dec;115(12):897–901.

Leonard R, Rees CJ, Belafsky P, Allen J. Fluoroscopic surrogate for pharyngeal strength: the pharyngeal constriction ratio (PCR). Dysphagia. 2011 March;26(1):13–7.

Rademaker AW, Pauloski BR, Logemann JA, Shanahan TK. Oropharyngeal swallow efficiency as a representative measure of swallowing function. J Speech Hear Res. 1994 April;37(2):314–25.

Yip H, Leonard R, Belafsky PC. Can a fluoroscopic estimation of pharyngeal constriction predict aspiration? Otolaryngol Head Neck Surg. 2006 Aug;135(2):215–7.

Chapter 8
Fluoroscopy and Dysphagia Outcome Measures

Clinicians have devised numerous instruments of analysis to standardize the interpretation of videofluoroscopic swallow studies (VFSS). Such instruments are useful to standardize VFSS analysis, quantify dysfunction, predict risk, and assess prognosis. The number of instruments that have been described is abundant. This chapter will review the Eating Assessment Tool (EAT-10), the Functional Oral Intake Scale (FOIS), the Penetration Aspiration Scale (PAS), the NIH-Swallowing Safety Score (NIH-SSS), the Modified Barium Swallow-Impairment Tool (MBSImP™©), and the Davis score.

Eating Assessment Tool (EAT-10)

Dysphagia is a symptom. Patients may have significant symptoms and no objective evidence of swallowing dysfunction or may have profound dysfunction with few symptoms. The EAT-10 is a validated measure of patient dysphagia symptoms (Table 8.1). It has proven successful in the determination of initial patient swallowing disability and in monitoring treatment efficacy. Some clinicians have suggested that an abnormal EAT-10 (≥ 2) can predict swallowing dysfunction and be used as a screening tool for aspiration risk. The instrument is given to every patient undergoing a VFSS at our center.

Functional Oral Intake Scale (FOIS)

The FOIS is an instrument utilized to document clinician recommendations for safe oral feeding based on instrumental findings and patient cofactors such as comorbidity, functional status, history of pneumonia and malnutrition, and individual accepted risk (Table 8.2). It is a 7-item scale ranging from no oral intake to total oral intake with no restrictions. The scale is useful to quantify the level of dietary restrictions recommended to a patient. It can help assess the initial level of patient disability and monitor treatment efficacy. The main utility of the FOIS is that it is

Table 8.1 Eating Assessment Tool-10

Item	0 = no problem				
	4 = severe problem				
1. I have lost weight due to my swallowing disorder.	0	1	2	3	4
2. I cannot eat out due to my swallowing disorder.	0	1	2	3	4
3. I exert too much effort swallowing while consuming liquid foods.	0	1	2	3	4
4. I exert too much effort swallowing while consuming solid foods.	0	1	2	3	4
5. I exert too much effort while taking pills.	0	1	2	3	4
6. I feel pain during swallowing.	0	1	2	3	4
7. My swallowing condition impacts the pleasure I take while eating.	0	1	2	3	4
8. Food gets held (stuck) in my throat while swallowing.	0	1	2	3	4
9. I cough while I eat.	0	1	2	3	4
10. Swallowing creates tension on me (swallowing stresses me out).	0	1	2	3	4

Table 8.2 Functional Oral Intake Scale

Level	Description
1	No oral intake
2	Tube dependence with minimal/inconsistent oral intake
3	Tube supplements with consistent oral intake
4	Total oral intake of a single consistency
5	Total oral intake of multiple consistencies requiring special preparation
6	Total oral intake with no special preparation, but must avoid specific foods or liquid items
7	Total oral intake with no restrictions.

a primary endpoint of the comprehensive dysphagia workup. Its limitation is that it does not reflect the etiology and pathophysiology of the swallowing dysfunction. It is necessary to distinguish between the FOIS recommended by the clinician and the actual diet consumed by the patient.

Penetration Aspiration Scale (PAS)

In 1996, Rosenbeck and colleagues developed the PAS to assign a numerical score to the degree of penetration and aspiration witnessed during VFSS. This eight-point scale assesses depth of bolus passage into the airway and the patient's response to the bolus (Table 8.3). A score of 1 represents the absence of penetration and increasing scores reflect more severe dysfunction to a maximum score of 8 that identifies silent aspiration (Figs. 8.1–8.6).

The initial development of the PAS evaluated the blinded assessment of VFSS from 15 patients with oropharyngeal dysphagia secondary to cerebrovascular accidents by four expert judges. Statistical analyses demonstrated good inter- and intra-judge correlation (kappa=0.96). The PAS is a gross measure of swallowing dysfunction and risk. The scale has been used to assess initial degree of swallowing dysfunction on VFSS and monitor response to therapy and surgery. The limitations of the PAS are that it does not elucidate swallowing physiology and has unreliable correlation with

Table 8.3 Penetration aspiration scale

Score	Description
1	Material does not enter the airway
2	Material enters the airway, remains above the vocal folds, and is ejected from the airway (Fig. 8.1)
3	Material enters the airway, remains above the vocal folds, and is not ejected from the airway
4	Material enters the airway, contacts the vocal folds, and is ejected from the airway (Fig. 8.2)
5	Material enters the airway, contacts the vocal folds, and is not ejected from the airway (Fig. 8.3)
6	Material enters the airway, passes below the vocal folds, and is ejected into the larynx or out of the airway (Fig. 8.4)
7	Material enters the airway, passes below the vocal folds, and is not ejected from the trachea despite effort (Fig. 8.5)
8	Material enters the airway, passes below the vocal folds, and no effort is made to eject (Fig. 8.6)

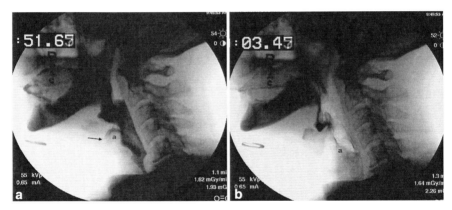

Fig. 8.1 Lateral fluoroscopic view of (**a**) penetration (*black arrow*) just over arytenoid complex, remaining above vocal folds. The subject reflexively coughs (**b**) and expels the material from the laryngeal vestibule. This represents a PAS score of 2

the degree of swallowing dysfunction (e.g., some patients with a normal PAS may have complete pharyngoesophageal segment (PES) obstruction and be dependent on nonoral tube feeding for 100 % of their nutritional requirements). These limitations have led other investigators to develop alternative rating instruments.

NIH Swallowing Safety Scale (NIH-SSS)

The NIH-SSS was developed to capture abnormalities involving pooling and lack of entry into the esophagus in the absence of penetration and aspiration. The NIH-SSS quantifies swallowing safety on the basis of seven observations from VFSS

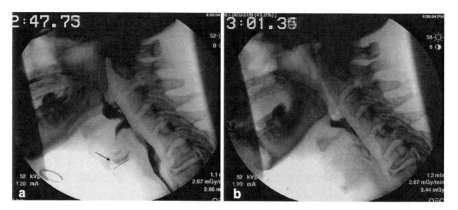

Fig. 8.2 Lateral fluoroscopic view of (**a**) penetration (*black arrow*) to vocal folds (*dotted black line*). Following a reflexive cough (**b**), the material is completely ejected from the laryngeal vestibule. This represents a PAS score of 4

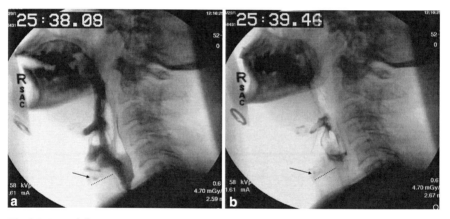

Fig. 8.3 Lateral fluoroscopic view demonstrating (**a**) penetration (*black arrow*) to level of vocal folds (*black dotted line*). An attempt is made at ejecting material (**b**) but contrast remains in laryngeal vestibule at level of vocal folds (*black arrow*). This represents a PAS score of 5

including residue, laryngeal penetration, aspiration, aspiration response, maximal esophageal entry, and multiple swallows (Table 8.4).

The NIH-SSS score is calculated from thin liquid trials. Higher scores indicate greater impairment. The advantages of the NIH-SSS are that it quantifies residue, penetration, aspiration, and entry into the esophagus. It has not, however, been rigorously validated nor has it been broadly accepted for clinical or scientific use.

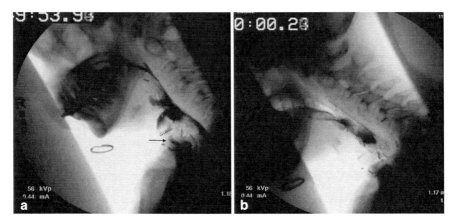

Fig. 8.4 Lateral fluoroscopic view showing (**a**) aspiration (*black arrow*), airway entry of material to level below the vocal folds (*black dotted line*). A cough (**b**) results in ejection from airway and near-complete clearance of laryngeal vestibule. This represents a PAS score of 6

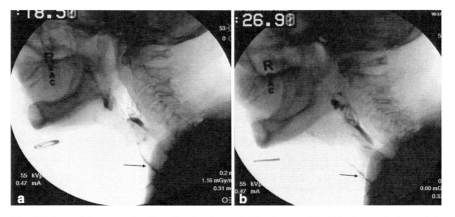

Fig. 8.5 Lateral fluoroscopic view showing (**a**) aspiration into trachea (*black arrow*). A cough is triggered (**b**) but material remains distal to vocal folds in trachea (*black arrow*). This represents a PAS score of 7

MBS Impairment Tool (MBSImP)

Developed by Dr. Martin-Harris, the MBSImP™© evaluates 17 parameters of swallowing including both physiologic and bolus flow measures (Table 8.5). Certified clinicians generate observation-based scores using the validated scoring protocol (Table 8.3). Further details regarding the protocol and guidelines for grading specific components are available in the MBSImP™© Guide (https://www.mbsimp.com/uploads/MBSImP-Guide.pdf). The advantages of the MBSImp are that it provides semiquantitative information of specific swallowing parameters and allows

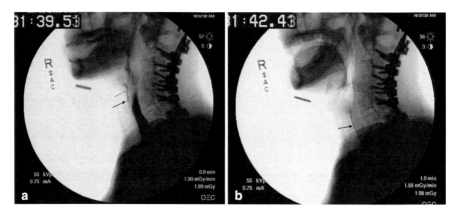

Fig. 8.6 Lateral fluoroscopic view showing (**a**) aspiration (*black arrow*) below the vocal folds (*black dotted line*) without triggering of a cough response (**b**) and passage of aspirated material into the more distal trachea (*black arrow*). This represents silent aspiration, or a PAS score of 8

Table 8.4 NIH-swallowing safety scale

Finding	Score
Residue in the vallecula	0 (absent) – 1 (present)
Penetration into vestibule from hypopharynx	0 (absent) – 1 (present)
Residue in the pyriform	0 (absent) – 1 (present)
Backup penetration from the pyriform into the laryngeal vestibule	0 (absent) – 1 (present)
Entry into upper esophagus	0 (100% entry) – 3 (no entry)
Aspiration	0 (absent) – 1 (present)

for the classification of diverse swallowing pathologies. The disadvantages are that it requires standardized and proprietary training and is time consuming to calculate and interpret.

Davis Score

At our center, we have developed a scoring system used to predict aspiration from a single, preswallow lateral fluoroscopic image. This Davis Score is simple to apply to a standard VFSS and provides the clinician with important clues to the likelihood of swallowing dysfunction (aspiration). Nine items (Table 8.6) representing risk factors for swallowing dysfunction make up the Davis Score. They were chosen by an interdisciplinary panel based on professional experience and face validity. The specific items evaluated are (1) dental health, (2) presence of mandibular hardware, (3) cervical spine abnormalities, (4) cervical spine hardware, (5) epiglottic abnormality, (6) thickening of the posterior pharyngeal wall, (7) subjective assessment of an enlarged pharyngeal area, (8) presence of tracheotomy tube, and (9) surgical clips in the neck.

Table 8.5 MBSImP scoring protocol

Parameter	Scoring
Lip closure	0: no escape of bolus between lips
	1: interlabial escape, but no progression to anterior lip
	2: escape from the interlabial space or lateral juncture with no extension beyond the vermillion border of the lower lip
	3: escape to the mid chin
	4: profuse spilling or escape of even small amounts beyond the mid chin through open lips
Hold position/Tongue control	0: normal
	1: bolus goes to either or both of the lateral sulci or the floor of the mouth, or is spread diffusely throughout the oral cavity
	2: any portion less than half of the bolus passes through the tongue-palate seal
	3: more than half of the bolus enters the pharynx
Bolus preparation/Mastication	0: timely and efficient chewing and mashing
	1: slow and prolonged chewing and mashing, but complete recollection or formation of the bolus is achieved
	2: the bolus is not formed and pieces remain in the oral cavity after the initial swallow
	3: minimal chewing and mashing with a majority of the bolus remaining unchewed
Bolus transport/lingual motion	0: normal
	1 (delay): prolonged holding followed by relatively normal movement
	2 (slow): seemingly weak tongue movement that progresses in a productive, posterior-ward motion
	3: slow and repetitive
	4: minimal or no observable movement
Oral residue	0: no barium remaining in the oral cavity
	1: trace residue resembles an outline of coated structures
	2: amount remaining in oral cavity is sufficient to extract or "scoop"
	3: more than half of the original bolus (majority) remains in the oral cavity
	4: minimal or no clearance of the bolus from the oral cavity
Initiation of pharyngeal swallow	0: bolus head at posterior angle of ramus and back of tongue at the first sign of hyoid excursion
	1: bolus head at the valleculae at the time of first hyoid excursion
	2: bolus head at the posterior laryngeal surface of the epiglottis at first onset of hyoid excursion
	3: bolus head in the pyriform sinus at the time of first hyoid excursion
	4: no appreciable initiation at any bolus location
Soft palate elevation	0: no bolus between soft palate and pharyngeal wall
	1: trace column of contrast or air between the soft palate and pharyngeal wall
	2: escape of contrast material to the level of the nasopharynx
	3: escape of contrast material that progress to the level of the nasal cavity
	4: escape of contrast material progressing to the level of the nostril

Table 8.5 (continued)

Parameter	Scoring
Laryngeal elevation	0: full superior movement of the thyroid cartilage that results in complete approximation of the arytenoids to the epiglottis petiole
	1: partial superior movement of the thyroid cartilage resulting in partial approximation of the arytenoids to the epiglottic petiole
	2: minimal superior movement of the thyroid cartilage resulting in minimal approximation of the arytenoids to the epiglottic petiole
	3: no superior movement of the thyroid cartilage and no approximation of the arytenoids to the epiglottic petiole
Anterior hyoid motion	0: complete anterior hyoid movement
	1: partial anterior movement of the hyoid bone
	2: no anterior movement of the hyoid bone
Epiglottic movement	0: complete inversion of the epiglottis
	1: movement of the epiglottis to a horizontal position with no progression beyond the horizontal position (or inferior movement without reaching a horizontal position)
	2: minimal movement of the epiglottis
Laryngeal closure	0: complete laryngeal vestibule closure with no air or contrast in the laryngeal vestibule
	1: narrow column of air or contrast in the laryngeal vestibule
	2: wide column of air or contrast in the laryngeal vestibule
Pharyngeal stripping wave	0: full wave of contraction from the level of the nasopharynx continuing to the level of the PES
	1: diminished wave along any portion of the posterior pharyngeal wall
	2: complete absence with no notable wave, often represented by a relatively straight line along the posterior pharyngeal wall
Pharyngeal contraction	0: symmetrical and complete contraction of the pharynx
	1: incomplete contraction
	2: unilateral bulging of one pharyngeal wall
	3: bilateral bulging of the both pharyngeal walls
PES opening	0: relatively straight edges through the segment with no appreciable narrowing from pharynx to proximal esophagus
	1: partial distention/partial duration with partial obstruction to flow while maintaining opening long enough for most of the bolus to pass
	2: minimal distention/minimal duration with marked obstruction resulting in resistance to bolus passage
	3: absence of PES opening and no bolus clearance
Tongue base retraction	0: complete retraction resulting in merging of tongue base with superior and middle posterior pharyngeal wall
	1: trace column of contrast that resembles an outline made with a fine tip pen between the tongue base and posterior pharyngeal wall
	2: narrow column of air or contrast between the tongue base and posterior pharyngeal wall
	3: wide column of air or contrast between the tongue base and posterior pharyngeal wall
	4: no appreciable movement of the tongue base

Table 8.5 (continued)

Parameter	Scoring
Pharyngeal residue	0: complete pharyngeal clearance
	1: trace residue of contrast within or on pharyngeal structures
	2: collection of residue within or on pharyngeal structures
	3: majority of contrast within or on pharyngeal structures
	4: minimal to no pharyngeal clearance
Esophageal clearance	0: complete esophageal clearance, even with coating
	1: mid-to-distal esophageal retention
	2: mid-to-distal esophageal retention with retrograde flow below the PES
	3: esophageal retention with retrograde flow through the PES
	4: minimal to no esophageal clearance

MBSImP modified barium swallow impairment tool, *PES* pharyngoesophageal segment

Table 8.6 Components of the Davis score

Site	Abnormality	Score
Teeth	Missing > 50%	1
Mandible	Presence of hardware	1
Cervical spine	Malformation at C3–C6	1
Spinal hardware	Present	1
Epiglottis	Absent, thickened, or malpositioned	1
Posterior pharyngeal wall	Thickness > 1/4 vertebral body width at C3	1
Pharyngeal area	Enlarged	1
Airway	Presence of tracheostomy tube	1
Soft tissue	Presence of surgical clips	1

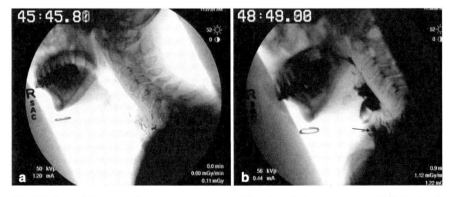

Fig. 8.7 Lateral fluoroscopic image demonstrates (**a**) enlarged pharyngeal area, ill-defined epiglottis, and surgical clips yielding a Davis Score of 3. (**b**) The patient experiences silent aspiration (*black arrow*) during a 10cc swallow trial

A score of one is given when an abnormality exists for a given parameter and zero if normal or does not meet criteria for abnormal. A Davis Score of two or greater predicted an individual was nearly seven times more likely to aspirate during the

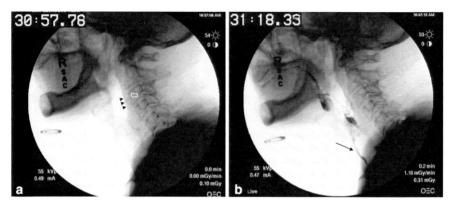

Fig. 8.8 Lateral fluoroscopic image demonstrates (**a**) an edentulous mandible and maxilla, thickened epiglottis, enlarged pharyngeal area and thickened posterior pharyngeal wall (*black arrowheads*) at C3 yielding a Davis score of 4. (**b**) On a 3cc trial, the patient exhibits silent aspiration (*black arrow*)

VFSS when compared to those with a Davis Score of less than two (unpublished) (Figs. 8.7 and 8.8). The scoring system has proven useful to assess aspiration risk before the administration of barium. The primary limitation is the lack of reproducibility for certain aspects of the scale.

Suggested Reading

Belafsky PC, Mouadeb DA, Rees CJ, Pryor JC, Postma GN, Allen J, Leonard RJ. Validity and reliability of the Eating Assessment Tool (EAT-10). Ann Otol Rhinol Laryngol. 2008 Dec;117(12):919–24.

Crary MA, Mann GD, Groher ME. Initial psychometric assessment of a functional oral intake scale for dysphagia in stroke patients. Arch Phys Med Rehabil. 2005 Aug;86(8):1516–20.

Rosenbek JC, Robbins JA, Roecker EB, Coyle JL, Wood JL. A penetration-aspiration scale. Dysphagia. 1996 Spring;11(2):93–98.

Ludlow CL, Humbert I, Saxon K, Poletto C, Sonies B, Crujido L. Effects of surface electrical stimulation both at rest and during swallowing in chronic pharyngeal Dysphagia. Dysphagia. 2007 Jan;22(1):1–10.

Martin-Harris B, Brodsky MB, Michel Y et al. MBS measurement tool for swallow impairment– MBSImp: establishing a standard. Dysphagia. 2008 Dec;23(4):392–405.

Chapter 9
Abnormal Oral and Pharyngeal Phase Fluoroscopy

A variety of abnormal findings can be identified on fluoroscopic evaluation of the oral cavity and pharynx. These first chambers of the aerodigestive tract are responsible for bolus preparation, formation, and containment as well as bolus propulsion, airway protection, and initial events of pharyngoesophageal segment (PES) opening (Chap. 4). Abnormalities are the result of a wide spectrum of causes that include congenital malformations, postsurgical status, radiation exposure, neuromuscular disorders, posttraumatic conditions, chronic systemic illness, neurodegenerative diseases and aging. The fluoroscopic finding of an oral or pharyngeal abnormality may not be solely responsible for a patient's dysphagia and comorbid fluoroscopic abnormalities of the pharyngeal and esophageal phases must be ruled out.

Abnormal Oral Fluoroscopy

The ability to feed and prepare a bolus from ingested material relies on adequate mouth opening, labial competence, masticatory forces, sufficient dentition as well as intact tongue and buccal motor and sensory function. There are a number of etiologies for limited jaw opening, or trismus (Table 9.1), and it is readily identified on VFSS. Limited mouth opening may significantly affect the ability to feed or prepare the bolus and may require diet modification, physical therapy, or surgical intervention. Additional fluoroscopic clues to disordered oral and masticatory function include the presence of mandibular hardware, missing dentition, and prosthodontics.

Intact tongue function is imperative for effective oral phase deglutition. The tongue participates in bolus formation, containment, posterior propulsion, and lingual-palatal valving (Chap. 4). Lingual hyperactivity may be seen during VFSS as excessive bolus preparation or tongue pumping (Fig. 9.1). Disordered tongue movement may indicate neurodegenerative disorder, most commonly Parkinson's disease, caution in the setting of a threatened airway, or anticipation of more distal swallowing impairment or obstruction. Tongue impairment may manifest on VFSS

P. C. Belafsky, M. A. Kuhn, *The Clinician's Guide to Swallowing Fluoroscopy,*
DOI 10.1007/978-1-4939-1109-7_9, © Springer Science+Business Media New York 2014

Table 9.1 Causes of trismus

Cause	Example
Inflammatory/Infectious	Pericoronitis
	Masticatory myositis
	Peritonsillar abscess
	Submucous fibrosis
Traumatic	Mandibular fracture
	Zygomatic arch fracture
Neoplasm	Parotid malignancy
	Retromolar trigone carcinoma
	Infratemporal fossa tumor
	Nasopharyngeal carcinoma
Medication	Phenothiazine
	Metachlopromide
	Tricyclic antidepressants
	Succinyl choline
Iatrogenic	Radiation therapy
	Mandibular osteoradionecrosis
	Chemotherapy (stomatitis)
Congenital	Altered development of condyle, coronoid process, glenoid fossa, or zygomatic arch
TMJ disorder	Ankylosis
	Arthritis synovitis
	Damaged meniscus
	Traumatic brain injury
	Muscular dystrophy
	ALS
	Multiple sclerosis
	Parkinson's disease

TMJ temporomandibular joint, *ALS* amyotrophic lateral sclerosis

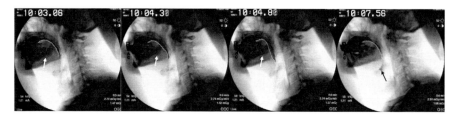

Fig. 9.1 Lateral fluoroscopic view demonstrates disordered oral preparatory phase. The oral tongue and tongue base (*white dotted line*) are pumping and there is bolus spillage into the oropharynx (*black arrow*) and the gingival buccal sulci (*white arrow*)

as oral spillage, early bolus loss into the oropharynx, and oral residue (Fig. 9.2). Common causes of lingual impairment (Table 9.2) include surgical resection (Fig. 9.3), muscular atrophy, weakness or immobility, and tethering. Fluoroscopic findings of lingual impairment are frequently accompanied by articulation difficulties and sometimes by labial incompetence.

Fig. 9.2 Lateral fluoroscopic view demonstrates abnormal oral residue coating the oral tongue (*white arrowheads*) and palate (*black arrowheads*). Also seen is residue within the vallecula (*black arrow*) and pharyngoesophageal segment (*white arrow*). Additionally, the patient has anterior cervical spinal hardware in place

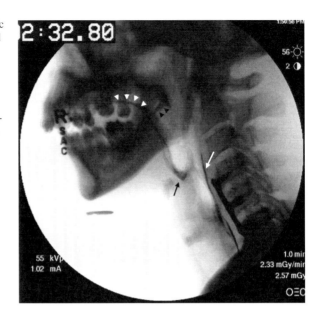

Table 9.2 Etiologies of oral tongue dysfunction

Etiology	Example
Neoplasm/Posttreatment	Intrinsic lingual tumor
	Other oral cavity tumor
	CNS tumor
	External beam radiation
	Glossectomy
Traumatic	Brain injury
	Facial trauma
	Hypoglossal nerve injury
Neurologic	Stroke
	Parkinson's disease
	Multiple sclerosis
	Cerebral palsy
	Muscular dystrophy
	Pseudobulbar palsy
	ALS
Congenital	Ankyloglossia
	Macroglossia
	Trisomy 21
	Pierre-Robin sequence
Autoimmune/Inflammatory	Fungal infection
	Xerostomia
	Sjogren's syndrome
	Myasthenia gravis
	Behcet's disease

CNS central nervous system, *ALS* amyotrophic lateral sclerosis

Fig. 9.3 Lateral fluoroscopic
view of an individual who
has had a near-total gloss-
ectomy for advanced head
and neck cancer. A small
remnant tongue is seen (*white
dotted line*) as is a palatal
prosthesis (*black arrow*). The
patient has poor oral bolus
control and early loss into the
oropharynx (*white arrow*)

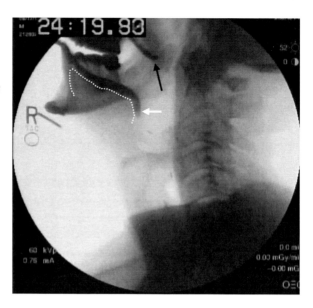

Abnormal Pharyngeal Fluoroscopy

The junction of the hard and soft palates and circumvallate papillae at the anterior base of tongue delineate the beginning of the oropharynx. The oropharynx
is critically important for safe and effective bolus propulsion and airway avoid-
ance (Chap. 4). Waldeyer's ring of lymphatic tissue includes the palatine, lingual,
and pharyngeal tonsils, and is susceptible to pathologic enlargement secondary to
acute infection, chronic inflammation, and neoplasm. Lymphatic abnormalities of
Waldeyer's ring can be visualized on VFSS (Fig. 9.4) and may result in dysfunction
due to odynophagia, obstruction, or restricted base of tongue mobility. Hypertrophy
of the lingual tonsil or base of tongue may be recognized on fluoroscopy as vallecular filing defects (Fig. 9.5). The vallecula may appear enlarged in individuals
with base of tongue defects or atrophy (Fig. 9.6). Such findings may be due to
neurologic processes, following surgical tongue base resection or radiation treatment to the pharynx. Physiologically, base of tongue deficiency may manifest as
early bolus loss, incomplete oropharyngeal clearing and residue, or penetration and
aspiration. Posteriorly, the vallecula is further bounded by the epiglottis, and irregularities of this structure are readily visualized on VFSS. Malformation, infection,
and neoplasms may appear as a blurred, enlarged, or widened epiglottis (Fig. 9.7).
Changes due to radiation therapy, surgery, or trauma may result in the appearance
of a shortened or absent epiglottis.

The pharynx is bounded posteriorly and laterally by pharyngeal wall composed
of the superior, middle, and inferior constrictors. The posterior pharyngeal wall

Fig. 9.4 Right anterior oblique fluoroscopic view with filling defect in the oropharynx (*white dashed line*) resulting from enlarged palatine tonsils

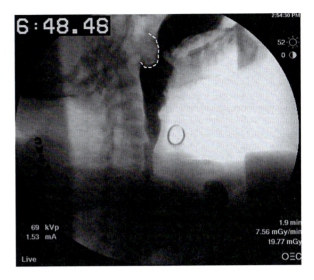

may become thickened and this is easily observed on VFSS (Fig. 9.8). Potential causes of posterior pharyngeal wall thickening include infectious processes, myositis, postradiation and surgical changes, and neoplasm. A thickened wall may impact the pharyngeal phase of swallowing by impeding the pharyngeal wave or preventing epiglottic inversion. Behind the posterior pharyngeal wall and the cervical esophagus are the vertebral bodies of the cervical spine. Its close proximity to the pharyngeal chamber means that cervical spine abnormalities may result in dysphagia. Commonly observed cervical spinal abnormalities include surgically placed hardware (Fig. 9.2), diffuse idiopathic skeletal hyperostosis (DISH) (Fig. 9.9), and

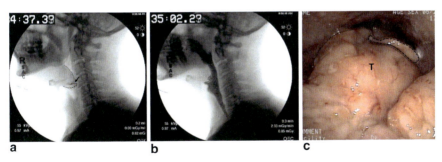

Fig. 9.5 Lateral fluoroscopic view (**a**) reveals a significantly enlarged tongue base (*black dotted line*) causing retroflexion of the epiglottis (*black hashed line*) and obliteration of the vallecula (*black arrow*). After ingestion of a 20cc bolus (**b**), the abnormal outline of the tongue is visible (*black dotted line*) as is the epiglottis (*black dashed line*). Endoscopy (**c**) shows significant enlargement of the tongue base (**T**) which makes contact with the epiglottis at rest (*black dashed line*)

Fig. 9.6 Lateral fluoroscopic view of a patient who had radiation treatment for a base-of-tongue tumor demonstrates notable tongue base atrophy (*white dotted line*). Pharyngeal residue (*black arrow heads*) in the vallecula and pyriforms is present. Also seen is hardware (*white arrows*) used to reconstruct the mandible after extirpation of osteoradionecrosis

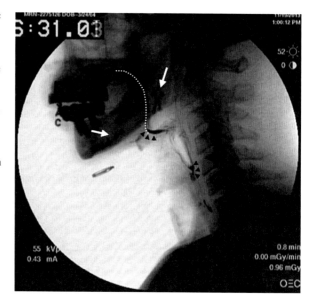

Fig. 9.7 A lateral fluoroscopic view shows a widened epiglottis (*black dotted line*)

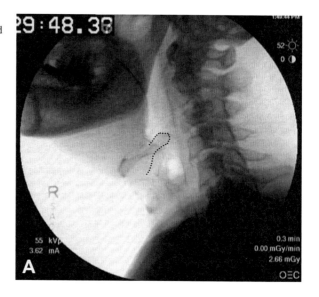

congenital curvatures (Fig. 9.10). The implications of such abnormalities on swallowing function are similar to those incurred with an enlarged posterior pharyngeal wall. Cervical hardware characteristically impairs epiglottic inversion, DISH may impede bolus flow, and severe scoliosis may result in an enlarged pharyngeal area and weakness. Chapter 10 includes a more comprehensive discussion of cervical osteophytes.

Commonly seen in the VFSSs of both normal and dysphagic individuals are lateral pharyngeal diverticula (LPD). They were first described in the late 19th

Fig. 9.8 A lateral fluoroscopic view of VFSS shows
a significantly enlarged posterior pharyngeal wall (*white
double arrow*). The thickness
should be between 0.3 to
0.4 cm at levels C3/4

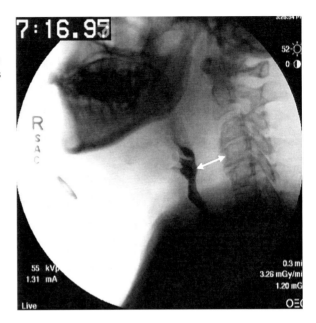

century and most contemporary clinicians distinguish pharyngeal diverticula from
pharyngoceles, or out-pouchings from the pharynx which have a characteristic radiographic appearance. On AP fluoroscopic views, pharyngeal diverticula have an
'ear' shape and are often attached to the pharynx by a more narrow neck (Fig. 9.11).
LPD are accepted as pulsion diverticula, occurring at areas of inherent weakness
in the pharyngeal wall including between the superior and middle pharyngeal

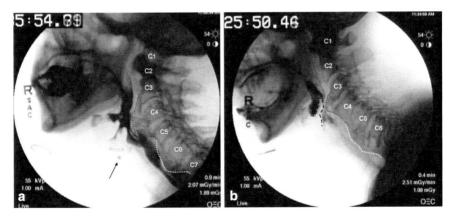

Fig. 9.9 Lateral views from fluoroscopic swallow studies of patients with diffuse idiopathic skeletal hyperostosis (DISH). In patient **a**, severe disease is seen from C3 to C5 (*black dotted line*)
and C5 to C7 (*white dotted line*), complete pharyngeal obliteration is not achieved and contrast
material is aspirated below the vocal folds (*black arrow*). Patient **b** has DISH most significantly
at C3 to C4 (*black dotted line*) and C4 to C7 (*white dotted line*). The degenerative spinal disease
prevents the epiglottis (*black dashed line*) from retroflexing

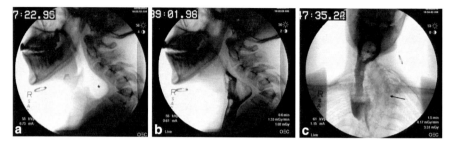

Fig. 9.10 Lateral fluoroscopic view (**a**) shows significant curvature of the cervical spine with resultant enlargement of the resting pharyngeal area (*black asterisk*). Upon swallowing (**b**) the pharynx does not completely constrict. Anterior-posterior fluoroscopy (**c**) reveals scoliosis of the cervical spine (*black asterisk*) and thoracic spine (*black arrow*) causing solid food dysphagia

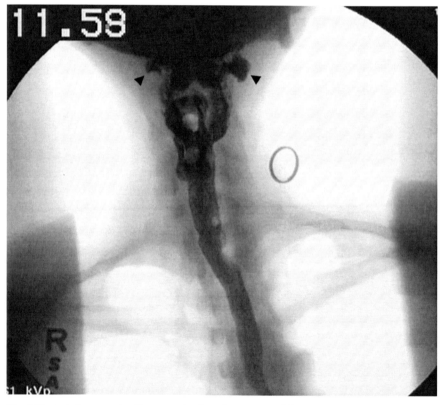

Fig. 9.11 Anterior-posterior fluoroscopic view demonstrates bilateral pharyngeal pulsion diverticula (*black arrowheads*)

constrictors, middle and inferior pharyngeal constrictors and thyrohyoid membrane. Radiographically, they appear at the inferior tonsillar fossa, level of the vallecula and pyriform sinus. Their diagnosis is most commonly made during fluoroscopic

	Cause	Example
Table 9.3 Etiologies of velopharyngeal insufficiency	Congenital	Cleft palate
		Submucosal cleft
		Trisomy 21
		Velocardiofacial syndrome
		Myotonic dystrophy
		Neurofibromatosis
	Iatrogenic	Tumor resection
		External beam radiation
		UPPP
		Adenoidectomy
		Tonsillectomy
	Neurologic	Cranial neuropathy
		Stroke
		Cerebral palsy
		Traumatic brain injury
		Muscular dystrophy
		ALS
		Multiple sclerosis
		Parkinson's disease

UPPP uvulopalatopharyngoplasty, *ALS* amyotrophic lateral sclerosis

evaluation of individuals with dysphagia though reports of endoscopically diagnosed LPD exist. If the LPD is suspected to be a source for an individual's swallowing complaints, treatment usually involves behavioral modifications though open and endoscopic surgical approaches have been described for cases with recidivistic symptoms. Among elderly patients, generalized decompensation, poor pulmonary status or neurologic dysfunction resulting in even small amounts of pharyngeal residue from LPD may place them at risk of aspiration sequelae.

Abnormal Velopharyngeal Fluoroscopy

Incomplete closure of the soft palate against the posterior pharyngeal wall results in velopharyngeal insufficiency (VPI). The palatopharyngeal valve is essential for proper articulation, prevention of nasopharyngeal and nasal reflux, and generation of proximal pharyngeal pressure to propel the travelling bolus forward. Impairment of this valve may result in nasopharyngeal regurgitation, hyper-nasal resonance in speech, profound dysphagia, and severe articulation dysfunction. There are various etiologies of palatopharyngeal valve dysfunction (PVD) (Table 9.3) including congenital, iatrogenic, neoplastic, and neurologic causes.

Videofluoroscopy assists the clinician in identifying and quantifying the presence of PVD and resultant VPI. On lateral VFSS, PVD is seen as the abnormal presence of air or contrast between the soft palate and pharyngeal wall while the bolus is transiting the oropharynx (Fig. 9.12a). The degree of VPI and the amount,

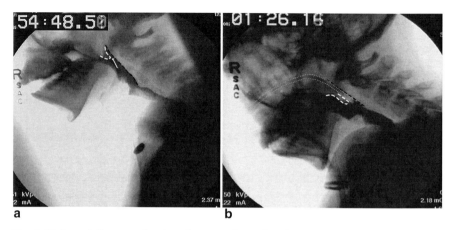

Fig. 9.12 Lateral fluoroscopic view demonstrating palatophary ngeal valve dysfunction and reflux of contrast (**a**, *white arrow*) between the soft palate (*white dashed line*) and the posterior pharyngeal wall (*black dashed line*). After sphincter pharyngoplasty (**b**), the apposition between the palate (*white dashed line*) and posterior pharyngeal wall (*black dashed line*) is improved, resorting competence to the palatopharyngeal valve. A temporary, post-operative nasogastric tube is visible (*grey dotted lines*).

if any, of nasopharyngeal or nasal reflux can be assessed which help guide treatment. Interventions for VPI include speech therapy with or without endoscopic biofeedback, palatal prostheses, and surgery (Fig. 9.12b). Choice of the surgical technique, pharyngoplasty, pharyngeal flap, or posterior pharyngeal wall augmentation, is often supported by endoscopic evaluation which helps differentiate lateral from anterior–posterior VPI.

Suggested Reading

Leonard R, Kendall C, editors. Dysphagia assessment and treatment planning: a team approach. 3rd edn. San Diego: Plural Publishing; 2013.

Shaker R., Belafsky PC, Postma GN, Easterling C, editors. Principles of deglutition: a multidisciplinary text for swallowing and its disorders. New York: Springer; 2012.

Shaker R, Belafsky PC, Postma GN, Easterling C, editors. Manual of diagnostic and therapeutic techniques for disorders of deglutition. New York: Springer; 2012.

Bodin IK, Lind MG, Arnande C. Free radial forearm flap reconstruction in surgery of the oral cavity and pharynx: surgical complications, impairment of speech and swallowing. Clin Otolaryngol Allied Sci. 1994 Feb;19(1):28–34.

Funk GF, Karnell LH, Christensen AJ. Long-term health-related quality of life in survivors of head and neck cancer. Arch Otolaryngol Head Neck Surg. 2012 Feb;138(2):123–33.

Gonzalez-Fernandez M, Daniels SK. Dysphagia in stroke and neurologic disease. Phys Med Rehabil Clin N Am. 2008 Nov;19(4):867–88.

Chapter 10
Abnormal Pharyngoesophageal Segment Fluoroscopy

The pharyngoesophageal segment (PES) is one of the only regions of the swallowing mechanism that is modifiable with therapy and surgery. A thorough knowledge of PES pathology is essential for all swallowing clinicians. The VFSS is the gold standard tool to diagnose PES dysfunction. A systematic approach to PES analysis ensures a comprehensive assessment of dysfunction (Table 10.1).

Evaluation of PES Fluoroscopic Anatomy

Initial evaluation of the PES begins with an evaluation of preswallow fluoroscopic anatomy. Abnormalities of the oral cavity, tongue base, epiglottis, pharyngeal area, posterior pharyngeal wall thickness, larynx and cricoid cartilages, and cervical spine may all influence PES function. Poor dentition, epiglottic and posterior pharyngeal wall edema, a low-lying larynx, pharyngeal dilation, and cervical osteophytes may all influence bolus transit through the PES. Irregularities in fluoroscopic anatomy are noted before barium is administered and the Davis Score is calculated (Chap. 8).

Evaluation of Laryngohyoid Elevation

The evaluation of the PES then continues with an assessment of hyoid and laryngeal elevation. PES opening relies on sufficient laryngohyoid elevation to lift the thyroid and cricoid cartilages off of the spine and prime the PES (Chap. 5—Phase II of UES opening). Although the subjective evaluation of laryngohyoid elevation is often attempted, such assessments are incapable of determining accurate and reproducible information, and objective measurements are essential (Chap. 7). Normal laryngohyoid elevation is gender, bolus size, and age dependent, with greater values measured for men, larger bolus sizes, and individuals older than 65 years of age. Normal elevation of the larynx and hyoid with a 20 cc bolus is 3.72 cm (+/−0.91) for men and 2.88 cm (+/−0.43) for women. A low-lying larynx will require more elevation to

P. C. Belafsky, M. A. Kuhn, *The Clinician's Guide to Swallowing Fluoroscopy*,
DOI 10.1007/978-1-4939-1109-7_10, © Springer Science+Business Media New York 2014

Table 10.1 Systematic evaluation of the PES in sequence

Evaluation of pre-swallow PES fluoroscopic anatomy
Evaluation of laryngohyoid elevation
Evaluation of pharyngeal contractility
Evaluation of PES opening
Evaluation of the posterior cricoid region
Evaluation of the posterior hypopharyngeal wall region
Evaluation of esophageal function

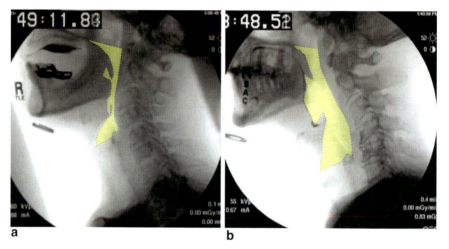

Fig. 10.1 Lateral fluoroscopic view displaying an individual with a normal (**a**) and dilated (**b**) pharyngeal area (*yellow highlighted region*)

raise it off of the spine. Tall individuals will also require a greater amount of elevation. Diminished laryngohyoid elevation will have a direct and diminutive influence on PES opening. After the assessment of laryngohyoid elevation, the systematic evaluation proceeds with the evaluation of pharyngeal contractility.

Evaluation of Pharyngeal Contractility

A pharynx that does not contract effectively will not have the ability to exert sufficient pressure on a bolus to distend the PES and allow its passage into the esophagus (Chap. 5—Phase III of UES opening). The fluoroscopic assessment of pharyngeal contractility begins with an evaluation of pharyngeal area. Pharyngeal area is assessed at rest while the administered bolus is held in the mouth (Fig. 10.1a, b). A dilated pharynx frequently does not contract efficiently and is a risk factor for aspiration (Fig. 10.2). Inter-rater reproducibility for the subjective determination of fluoroscopic pharyngeal dilation by established experts is only 72 % making objective

Fig. 10.2 Lateral
fluoroscopic view displaying
a dilated pharynx at rest
(*red dotted line*) and
aspirated barium (*red arrows*)

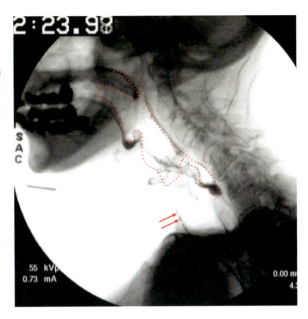

measurement of this parameter essential. Pharyngeal contractility on fluoroscopy is objectively assessed with the calculation of the pharyngeal constriction ratio (PCR). The PCR is a validated surrogate measure of pharyngeal strength on fluoroscopy (Chap. 7). It is defined as the maximal pharyngeal area during passage of a bolus divided by the pharyngeal area with the bolus held in the oral cavity. The PCR is calculated on the largest bolus that can be safely administered (10 or 20 cc). As pharyngeal constriction diminishes the PCR increases. A weak pharynx that has an elevated PCR on fluoroscopy will have a decreased ability to distend the larynx off of the spine during deglutition (Chap. 5—Phase III of UES opening) and PES opening will be reduced. PCR is also associated with age as the senile pharynx becomes thin and dilated. A PCR greater than 0.25 is associated with a threefold increase in the prevalence of aspiration.

Evaluation of PES Opening

After the assessment of laryngohyoid elevation and pharyngeal contractility, the systematic assessment proceeds with the determination of the opening dimensions of the PES. The PES is a 3–4-cm-long region of high pressure. The narrowest cross section of this region is referred to as "PES opening" and is measured during passage of the largest swallowed liquid barium bolus in the lateral and AP fluoroscopic views (Figs. 10.3 and 10.4). This measurement represents the area of greatest constraint to bolus flow. If lingual or pharyngeal weakness or diminished airway protection restrict the amount of barium that can be safely administered to the

Fig. 10.3 Lateral fluoroscopic view displaying region of PES opening measurement (*double white arrow*). Also visible is a cricopharyngeus muscle bar (*asterisk*) and a jet effect (*J*) below the bar. A jet is a pocket of air that is created from the flow of barium beneath a region of obstruction

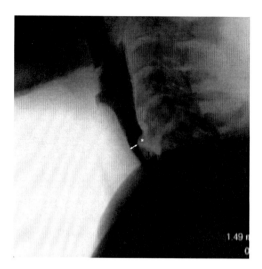

Fig. 10.4 Anterior-posterior fluoroscopic view displaying region of PES-opening measurement (*double white arrow*)

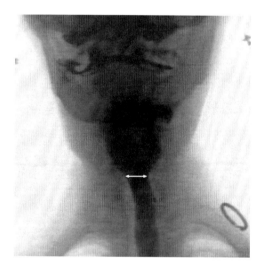

patient, the assessment of accurate PES opening will be limited. Normative data for objective PES opening are influenced by age, gender, and bolus size and are available for young and elderly (>65 years) male and female persons for both 10 and 20 cc boluses (Chap. 7). Normal mean PES opening with a 20 cc bolus is 0.90 cm (+/−0.28) for a person<65 and 0.80 cm (+/−0.20) for an individual>65 years of age. Diminished PES opening can be secondary to diminished elevation, poor lingual and pharyngeal constriction, decreased compliance as occurs with radiation induced stenosis, cricopharyngeus muscle (CPM) dysfunction, web, and neoplasm. After the assessment of PES opening, the systematic evaluation of the PES proceeds with an assessment of the posterior cricoid (PC) region.

Fig. 10.5 Cricopharyngeal web on lateral fluoroscopic view. The web is protruding off of the posterior rim of the cricoid cartilage (*black arrow*). The cricopharyngeus muscle (*asterisk*) is tethered to the web severely reducing opening of the upper esophageal sphincter

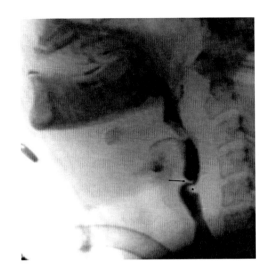

Evaluation of the PC Region

The PC region is defined as the area immediately adjacent to the posterior rim of the cricoid cartilage on the anterior wall of the esophageal inlet. It is differentiated from the posterior hypopharyngeal region, which is the adjacent region on the dorsal side of the esophageal inlet (Fig. 5.11). Findings of the PC region include cricoid impressions, plications, and webs. Findings of the posterior hypopharyngeal region include CPM bars and diverticuli. Precise fluoroscopic evaluation of these regions requires a large (20 cc) bolus to adequately distend the larynx and cricoid off of the spine. The inability to consume a large bolus due to lingual or pharyngeal weakness or unsafe airway protection will have a significant impact on the ability to identify PES opening and pathology.

Although not pathologic, the presence of a PC plication or PC impression is noted (Figs. 5.12 and 5.13). Cricopharyngeal webs are pathologic and are present in 14 % of dysphagic persons undergoing a VFSS. Large webs are readily visible and can tether the CPM and give the appearance of a CPM bar (Figs. 10.5 and 10.6). It is essential to identify a web that is tethering the CPM because treatment with simple dilation is usually curative and a more invasive CPM myotomy is unnecessary. Small webs do not tether the CPM and are easily missed. They can only be visualized with the administration of a large barium bolus, a high index of suspicion, and stop-motion analysis of video with a minimum capture rate of 30 frames per second (fps) (Figs. 5.14, 10.7). The addition of a 13 mm barium tablet to the VFSS helps identify webs that reduce the pharyngoesophageal lumen to 13 mm or less but does not assist with the recognition of smaller webs. Small cricopharyngeal webs are one of the most commonly missed fluoroscopic abnormalities in persons with solid food dysphagia. After the PC region is assessed, attention is then turned towards pathology of the posterior hypopharyngeal region.

Fig. 10.6 Cricopharyngeal web visualized on endoscopy. The web (*white arrows*) is tethering the cricopharyngeus muscle (CPM), severely reducing opening of the upper esophageal sphincter. Cricopharyngeal webs are not usually visible on endoscopy. This view was obtained by stop-motion frame-by-frame analysis during an eructation

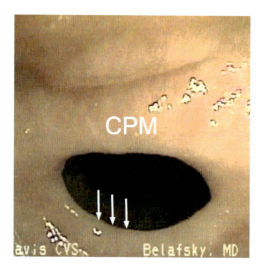

Fig. 10.7 Small cricopharyngeal web (*white arrows*) on right anterior oblique view. There is a small jet (*J*) effect

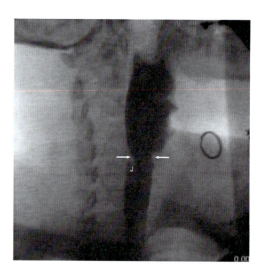

Evaluation of the Posterior Hypopharyngeal Wall Region

The most common abnormality of the posterior hypopharyngeal region is the presence of a CPM bar. CPM bars are due to a hypertrophied or poorly relaxing CPM and are not necessarily pathologic. They are seen in 30% of normal elderly individuals without dysphagia. We differentiate CPM bars into non-obstructing (NOB), moderately obstructing (MOB), and severely obstructing bars (SOB) based on the degree of minimum PES opening observed with a 20 cc bolus. A NOB (Fig. 10.8) is defined as the presence of a CPM bar with normal PES opening (>0.60 cm). A MOB is defined as the presence of a CPM bar with PES opening between 0.30 and

Fig. 10.8 A nonobstructing cricopharyngeus muscle bar (NOB) in the lateral fluoroscopic view (*asterisk*). Upper esophageal sphincter opening (*double-headed white arrow*) is normal (>0.60 cm). There is a small jet effect (*J*)

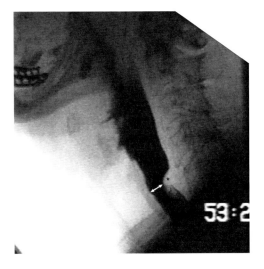

0.60 cm (Fig 10.9) and a SOB exists when PES opening is<0.30 cm (Fig. 10.10). Dysphagia is a symptom and dependent on patient-specific factors such as dentition, diet, chewing habits, and degree of visceral sensitivity. We have encountered patients with NOBs who experience significant dysphagia and patients with SOBs who experience little if any dysphagia. Association of objective findings on VFSS with subjective symptoms as documented on the Eating Assessment Tool (EAT-10) is necessary to formulate a patient-specific treatment strategy.

CPM bars may also be protective and a fluoroscopic evaluation of the esophageal phase of deglutition is essential to evaluate the protective function of the CPM. Esophageal webs, rings, hernias, strictures, and ineffective esophageal motility may all influence PES function. Esophageal stasis and backflow is associated with hypertrophy of the CPM and the development of CPM bars. The clinician must differentiate enlarged CPM bars that protect the airway against the regurgitation of esophageal and gastric contents from CPM bars that obstruct anterograde bolus transit through the PES. Although NOBs may cause the symptom of dysphagia, we do not consider CPM bars pathologic on fluoroscopy until the objective measurement of PES opening is abnormal (< 0.6 cm). Some CPM bars are both protective and pathologic and the clinician must decide if the pathologic obstruction caused by the bar is more significant to patient health than the benefit of the protective function of the muscle. Causes of esophageal dysfunction such as stricture, hernia, and achalasia must be addressed before consideration is given to surgery (myotomy) that would affect the ability of the CPM to protect the airway (Figs. 10.11 and 10.12). If esophageal function cannot be significantly improved, the clinician may consider more conservative PES treatment such as dilation instead of a more invasive myotomy. In our experience, dilation causes less detriment to the protective function of the PES than myotomy. A series of three dilations separated by 4–6 weeks is often recommended for CPM bars with significant PES obstruction.

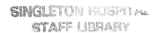

Fig. 10.9 A moderately obstructing cricopharyngeus muscle bar (MOB) in the lateral fluoroscopic view (*asterisk*). Upper esophageal sphincter opening is reduced and between 0.30 and 0.60 cm (*double-headed white arrow*). The hypopharynx is dilated above the MOB (*small black arrows*) giving the appearance of a small Zenker diverticulum. There is penetration of barium over the arytenoid cartilage (AC) into the laryngeal vestibule to the level of the true vocal folds (*long black arrows*)

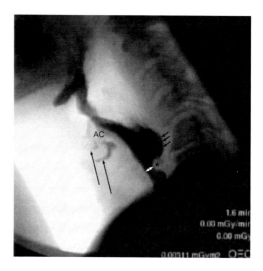

Fig. 10.10 A severely obstructing cricopharyngeus muscle bar (SOB) in the lateral fluoroscopic view (*asterisk*). Upper esophageal sphincter opening is reduced (*long black arrow*) and less than 0.30 cm. The hypopharynx is dilated above the SOB (*short black arrows*) giving the appearance of a small Zenker diverticulum

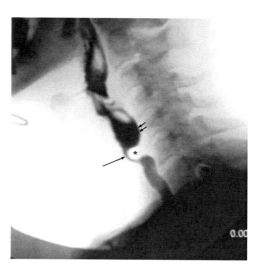

The effect of PES obstruction on the pharynx must also be considered before determining the necessity of PES surgery. A lumen that contracts against obstruction will become dilated and weakened over time. As PES opening becomes progressively reduced, pharyngeal area becomes increasingly dilated (Figs. 10.9 and 10.10). There is a linear association between the degree of PES obstruction and the resultant pharyngeal dilation (Fig. 10.13). Pharyngeal dilation and weakness are poorly reversible, even after PES obstruction has been relieved. Therefore, evidence of PES obstruction must be assessed within the context of pharyngeal function. A mildly obstructing CPM bar without evidence of pharyngeal dilation or weakness may be treated more conservatively (dilation) or even observed with yearly fluoroscopic

Fig. 10.11 Obstructing cricopharyngeus muscle bar (*asterisk*) in a person with an esophageal stricture and a large hiatal hernia (Fig. 10.12)

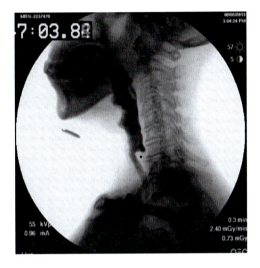

Fig. 10.12 A large hiatal hernia (*red arrowheads*) and an esophageal stricture (*black arrow*) in a person with an obstructing cricopharyngeus muscle bar (Fig. 10.11). *Red arrows* diaphragmatic hiatus

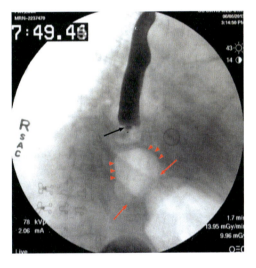

follow-up (*swallow-up* VFSS) to monitor for progression. A moderately or severely obstructing CPM bar with evidence of pharyngeal dilation and weakness is treated more aggressively (dilation/myotomy) to prevent further irreversible deterioration of pharyngeal function. A person who presents with profound aspiration secondary to pharyngeal weakness may not be able to safely consume sufficient quantities of barium to adequate identify PES pathology that may be causative in the pharyngeal dilation and swallowing dysfunction. This is one of the most significant limitations of the VFSS.

There is a region of anatomic weakness with a lack of muscular support between the inferior pharyngeal constrictor and the CPM known as Killian's dehiscence.

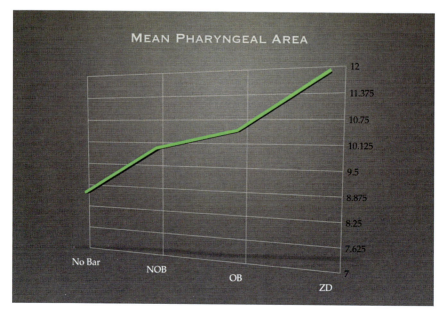

Fig. 10.13 The association between degree of obstruction at the pharyngoesophageal segment (*PES*) and mean pharyngeal area. Pharyngeal area displays a linear increase as the PES obstruction progresses along the continuum from no cricopharyngeus muscle (*CPM*) bar to a nonobstructing bar (*NOB*) to an obstructing CPM bar (*OB*) to a Zenker diverticulum (*ZD*)

A Zenker diverticulum (ZD) forms when the hypopharynx dilates and hypopharyngeal mucosa and submucosa herniate through Killians's dehiscence and form a pouch (Fig. 10.14). Hypopharyngeal diverticuli must be differentiated from lateral pharyngeal diverticuli that are frequently asymptomatic and form in areas of inherent pharyngeal weakness (Chap. 9). The lateral fluoroscopic view is essential for the evaluation of ZD. It affords the assessment of PES opening, stasis, regurgitation, pharyngeal dilation and strength, and airway protection. The length of the diverticulum is also measured on lateral view from the tip of the obstructing CPM to the posterior base of the diverticulum (Fig. 10.14). The size of the ZD is important in planning an approach for surgical management. It is essential to increase the kVp of the fluoroscopy unit and penetrate through the soft tissue of the shoulder in the lateral view to effectively visualize bolus transit through the PES into the cervical esophagus. Failure to do so can lead to inaccurate diagnosis and inappropriate management. The anterior–posterior view allows the clinician to assess the laterality of the ZD and visualize the degree of residue within the pouch (Fig. 10.15). It may also help identify ZD that were missed on lateral view because of inadequate penetration of radiation through the soft tissue of the shoulder. It is also essential to evaluate the esophageal phase of swallowing to rule out comorbid esophageal pathology. The pathophysiology of ZD is considered to be dilation and herniation of the hypopharynx caused by years of constriction against a poorly compliant CPM.

Fig. 10.14 A lateral fluoroscopic view of a 2.3-cm Zenker diverticulum. The size of the ZD (*black arrows*) is measured from the tip of the obstructing cricopharyngeus muscle (*red arrowhead*) to the posterior base of the ZD (*white arrow*). The lumen of the esophageal inlet is severely narrowed and reduced to 1 mm (*red arrows*)

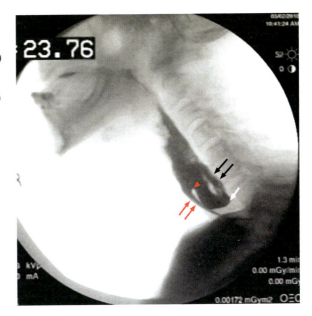

Fig. 10.15 An anterior-posterior view of the Zenker diverticulum in Fig. 10.14. The diverticulum is broad and bilobed (*red arrowheads*)

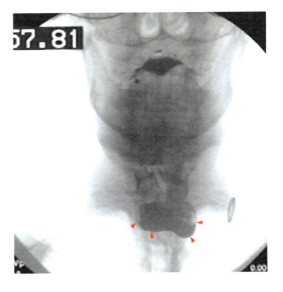

A familial preponderance of ZD has been reported and suggests a congenital weakness of Killian's dehiscence as a potential cofactor in diverticulum development.

It can be difficult to assess the PES after ZD surgery. After an open resection of the diverticulum and CPM myotomy, the region of the PES should appear nearly normal (Figs. 10.16a and b). Endoscopic stapling and laser diverticulotomy, however, have become the preferred approaches to ZD treatment. The endoscopic pro-

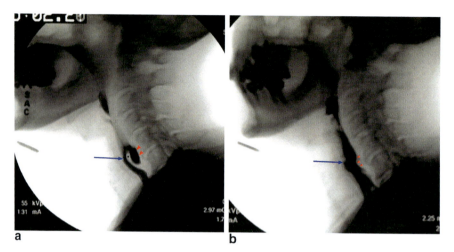

Fig. 10.16 A lateral fluoroscopic view of a Zenker diverticulum (ZD) before (**a**) and after (**b**) open diverticulectomy and cricopharyngeus muscle (CPM) myotomy. Preoperatively (Fig. 10.16a), the CPM is significantly enlarged (*asterisk*) and UES opening is severely reduced (*blue arrow*). There is a 1.7-cm ZD (*red arrowheads*). Postoperatively (Fig. 10.16b), the ZD is completely gone. There are slight postsurgical changes where the remnant of the CPM is (*red arrowheads*) and UES opening has returned to normal (*blue arrow*)

cedures do not remove the diverticulum. The surgeries improve bolus flow by dividing the CPM and party wall between the ZD and esophagus. After successful surgery, the source of obstruction is relieved and the diverticulum is free to drain into the esophagus without regurgitating into the hypopharynx. To the untrained clinician, fluoroscopy after an effective endoscopic procedure will appear similar to the preoperative examination. The clinician must not focus on the persistence of the diverticulum postoperatively but must assess the increase in PES opening and the decrease in pharyngeal dilation and hypopharyngeal regurgitation (Figs. 10.17a–d).

A ZD, by definition, occurs above a constricting CPM. Another type of hypopharyngeal diverticulum may occasionally be seen below the level of the CPM. Killian–Jamieson (KJ) diverticuli herniate through an area of weakness between the CPM superiorly and the longitudinal esophageal muscle inferiorly (Fig. 10.18). They are rare and it is essential that the clinician be able to differentiate between a ZD and a KJ diverticulum as treatment approaches differ significantly. KJ diverticuli are often asymptomatic. Because they may represent a serendipitous finding, it is essential to perform a full esophageal evaluation to rule out alternative causes of a person's dysphagia such as esophageal dysmotility or esophagitis. Large KJ diverticuli can occasionally become symptomatic and an open surgical approach may be necessary to excise the pouch. Unlike ZD where a CPM myotomy is essential to successful treatment, it is frequently not necessary to perform a CPM myotomy in patients with a KJ diverticulum. In fact, the CPM may be protective and it may be more appropriate to perform a myotomy of the esophageal longitudinal muscle distal to the diverticulum.

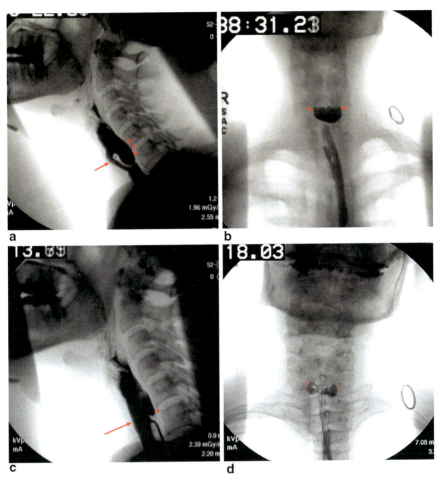

Fig. 10.17 Lateral and anterior posterior fluoroscopic views before (**a** and **b**) and after (**c** and **d**) endoscopic staple-assisted Zenker diverticulotomy. Preoperatively (Figs. 10.17a and 10.17b), the cricopharyngeus muscle (CPM) is significantly enlarged (*blue asterisk*) and UES opening is severely reduced (*red arrow*). There is a 2.0-cm Zenker diverticulum (ZD) (*red arrowheads*). Postoperatively (Figs. 10.17c and 10.17d), UES opening is significantly improved and is now within normal limits (*red arrow*). The ZD can still be visualized in both the lateral and anterior posterior views (*red arrowheads*). This is a normal fluoroscopic appearance of an endoscopic diverticulotomy with a successful outcome

Cervical osteophytes are another cause of pathology in the posterior hypopharyngeal region. Cervical osteophytes are common and may be present in more than 50% of asymptomatic elderly individuals. The vast majority of cervical osteophytes are asymptomatic. Rarely, however, they can enlarge and cause compressive symptoms during swallowing (Figs. 10.19 and 10.20). Two of the most common causes of pathologic anterior cervical osteophytes are diffuse idiopathic skeletal hyperostosis (DISH) and ankylosing spondylitis (AS). DISH, also known as Forestier's disease,

Fig. 10.18 An anterior-posterior fluoroscopic view of a Killian-Jamieson (KJ) diverticulum. The diverticulum (*red arrows*) can be seen below the cricopharyngeus muscle (*asterisk*)

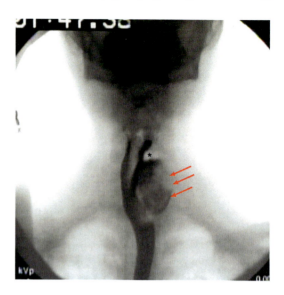

Fig. 10.19 Lateral fluoroscopic view of a person with diffuse idiopathic skeletal hyperostosis (DISH) and an obstructing cervical osteophyte (*asterisk*) distorting the epiglottis and causing profound swallowing dysfunction

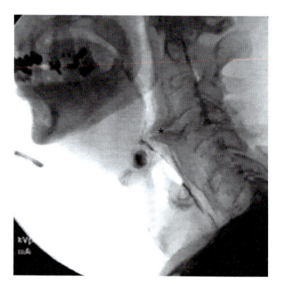

involves calcification and ossification within the anterior longitudinal ligament of at least four contiguous vertebral bodies. Dysphagia in DISH can be secondary to mechanical obstruction caused by the osteophytes or from posterior pharyngeal or hypopharyngeal inflammation with edema and fibrosis due to chronic irritation. Anti-inflammatory medication may improve dysphagia early in the disease process. It is essential to exclude alternative pathology that may be responsible for an individual's swallowing complaints and assess the integrity of the pharynx. Pharyngeal dilation and weakness may develop as a consequence of prolonged bony obstruc-

Fig. 10.20 Endoscopic view of the pharynx displayed in Fig. 10.15. The osteophyte (*asterisk*) is obscuring the laryngeal vestibule and obstructing the airway

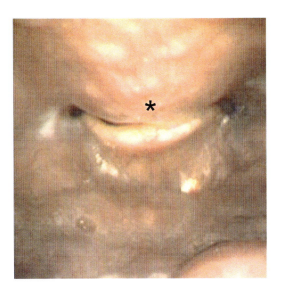

tion in the hypopharynx and the benefit of surgical excision of the osteophytes may depend on the degree of residual pharyngeal strength.

After a thorough evaluation of the posterior hypopharyngeal region has been performed, the systematic evaluation of the PES involves an evaluation of esophageal function.

Evaluation of Esophageal Function

Our experience suggests that esophageal pathology (hiatal hernia, esophageal dysmotility, reflux, stricture) may be more frequent in patients with CPM dysfunction and ZD. An esophageal evaluation is required to determine the protective nature of the CPM and rule out alternative esophageal pathology contributing to a person's dysphagia. We recommend a comprehensive videofluoroscopic esophagram in all persons with PES dysfunction to adequately establish a comprehensive treatment plan (Chaps. 3, 6, 11).

Suggested Reading

Allen J, White CJ, Leonard R, Belafsky PC. Effect of cricopharyngeus muscle surgery on the pharynx. Laryngoscope. 2010 Aug;120(8):1498–503.

Allen JE, White CJ, Leonard RJ, Belafsky PC. Posterior cricoid region fluoroscopic findings: the posterior cricoid plication. Dysphagia. 2011 Sep; 26(3):272–6.

Belafsky PC, Rees CJ, Allen J, Leonard RJ. Pharyngeal dilation in cricopharyngeus muscle dysfunction and Zenker diverticulum. Laryngoscope. 2010 May;120(5):889–94.

Fuller SC, Leonard R, Aminpour S, Belafsky PC. Validation of the pharyngeal squeeze maneuver. Otolaryngol Head Neck Surg. 2009 Mar;140(3):391–4.

Kendall KA, Leonard RJ, McKenzie S. Airway protection: evaluation with videofluoroscopy. Dysphagia. 2004 Spring;19(2):65–70.

Kuhn MA, Belafsky PC. Management of cricopharyngeus muscle dysfunction. Otolaryngol Clin North Am. 2013 Dec;46(6):1087–99.

Leonard R, Kendall KA, McKenzie S. Structural displacements affecting pharyngeal constriction in nondysphagic elderly and nonelderly adults. Dysphagia. 2004 Spring;19(2):133–41.

Leonard R, Kendall K, McKenzie S. UES opening and cricopharyngeal bar in nondysphagic elderly and nonelderly adults. Dysphagia. 2004 Summer;19(3):182–91.

Leonard R, Belafsky PC, Rees CJ. Relationship between fluoroscopic and manometric measures of pharyngeal constriction: the pharyngeal constriction ratio. Ann Otol Rhinol Laryngol. 2006 Dec;115(12):897–901.

Leonard R, Kendall C, editors. Dysphagia assessment and treatment planning: a team approach. 2nd edn. San Diego: Plural Publishing; 2007.

Leonard R, Belafsky P, McKenzie S. Pharyngeal adaptation in Zenker's diverticulum: the "faux pharyngoesophageal segment". Otolaryngol Head Neck Surg. 2008 Sep;139(3):424–8.

Leonard R, Rees CJ, Belafsky P, Allen J. Fluoroscopic surrogate for pharyngeal strength: the pharyngeal constriction ratio (PCR). Dysphagia. 2011 Mar;26(1):13–7.

Shaker R, Belafsky PC, Postma GN, Easterling C, editors. Principles of deglutition: a multidisciplinary text for swallowing and its disorders. New York: Springer; 2012.

Shaker R, Belafsky PC, Postma GN, Easterling C, editors. Manual of diagnostic and therapeutic techniques for disorders of deglutition. New York: Springer; 2012.

Yip H, Leonard R, Belafsky PC. Can a fluoroscopic estimation of pharyngeal constriction predict aspiration? Otolaryngol Head Neck Surg. 2006 Aug;135(2):215–7.

Chapter 11
Abnormal Esophageal Fluoroscopy

A focused but comprehensive dysphagia history is essential for accurate interpretation of the videofluoroscopic esophagram (VFE). In an ambulatory person with solid food dysphagia, an esophageal contribution to the swallowing complaint will be present in 60% of individuals. The most common causes of dysphagia in this population include esophagitis, pharyngoesophageal webs, ineffective esophageal motility (IEM), and Schatzki's rings. Esophageal strictures are less common in the era of widespread proton pump inhibitor use but are still prevalent. Although esophageal cancer is rare, it is essential for the clinician to identify subtle changes on fluoroscopy suggestive of this diagnosis. Persons with Barrett metaplasia have diminished esophageal sensitivity and are less likely to suffer from frequent heartburn. It is for this reason that most esophageal cancers present as obstructing dysphagia and not with persistent heartburn. The most concerning patient history is that of an individual that used to suffer from heartburn but now has weight loss and solid food dysphagia. The presence of odynophagia is also concerning and usually signifies more severe esophageal pathology. The localization of the swallowing complaint is important to elicit. An individual who points to the cervical region will have co-morbid esophageal dysfunction in 30%. Localization of the dysphagia to the chest indicates an esophageal etiology in the majority of cases. A history of head and neck cancer, radiation exposure, or oropharyngeal dysphagia of another etiology may influence the amount of barium administered during the esophagram. A systematic approach to the evaluation of VFE pathology ensures a comprehensive assessment of esophageal dysfunction (Table 11.1).

Evaluation of Pharyngoesophageal Segment (PES) Transit Abnormalities

The initial evaluation of the VFE begins with an assessment of transit through the pharyngoesophageal segment (PES). The presence of PES narrowing from cricopharyngeus muscle dysfunction (bar), web, stricture, or neoplasm is noted (Chap. 10). The right anterior oblique (RAO) view afforded by the VFE provides a unique and

P. C. Belafsky, M. A. Kuhn, *The Clinician's Guide to Swallowing Fluoroscopy,* 95
DOI 10.1007/978-1-4939-1109-7_11, © Springer Science+Business Media New York 2014

Table 11.1 Systematic evaluation of the videofluoroscopic esophagram in sequence

Evaluation of PES transit abnormalities

Evaluation of esophageal mucosal pathology

Evaluation of esophageal motility

Evaluation of obstructing esophageal pathology (web, ring, stricture)

Evaluation of diverticuli

Evaluation of hiatal hernia

Evaluation of gastroesophageal reflux

PES pharyngoesophageal segment

Fig. 11.1 A right anterior oblique view on videofluoroscopic esophagram of a small esophageal web (*red arrows*) that was missed on the lateral fluoroscopic view of a videofluoroscopic swallow study

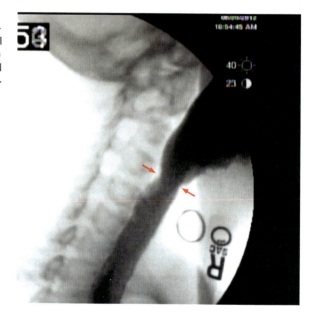

unobstructed view of PES anatomy and barium flow. Subtle pathology, such as a small cricopharyngeal web missed on lateral fluoroscopic view can be identified on the RAO view of the VFE (Fig. 11.1). After the PES is evaluated, the VFE evaluation proceeds with an assessment of esophageal mucosal pathology.

Evaluation of Esophageal Mucosal Pathology

The double contrast phase of the study highlights mucosal pathology that may otherwise be missed. The normal distended esophagus has a smooth homogenous contour (Fig. 11.2). Partially collapsed mucosal relief views may reveal mucosal changes signifying underlying pathology such as neoplasm or esophagitis (Figs. 11.3 and 11.4). The most common cause of esophagitis is gastroesophageal reflux (peptic

Fig. 11.2 Normal mucosal appearance of the distended esophagus (*red arrows*)

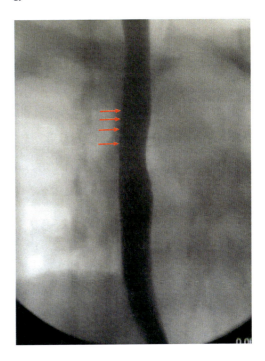

esophagitis). Esophageal inflammation and edema can result in a nodular appearance on VFE (Fig. 11.4). The VFE is poorly sensitive to diagnose mild esophagitis. Infectious esophagitis is much less common than reflux esophagitis. The most common cause of infectious esophagitis is candida. Candida esophagitis results in a characteristic granular appearance on VFE (Figs. 11.5 and 11.6). Other much less common causes of infectious esophagitis include herpes and cytomegalovirus (CMV) (Figs. 11.7 and 11.8). Eosinophillic esophagitis (EoE) is a rapidly increasing atopic cause of solid food dysphagia. Although the diagnosis of EoE is made on endoscopic biopsy displaying > 20 eosinophils per high-power field, there is a characteristic appearance on VFE that is highly suggestive of EoE. The distinguishing finding is that of segmental esophageal strictures giving the appearance of a corrugated or ringed esophagus (Figs. 11.9 and 11.10). In the absence of a ringed esophagus, a small caliber esophagus also suggests the presence of fibrotic narrowing secondary to the eosinophilic infiltrate (Fig. 11.11).

An evaluation of the mucosa concludes with an assessment of the esophageal mucosal folds. The longitudinal mucosal folds of the esophagus are normally thin, straight, and less than 2 mm in width. Prominent mucosal folds indicate esophageal inflammation and suggest the presence of esophagitis (Figs. 11.12 and 11.13). Esophageal varices produce an irregular, serpiginous, almost colonic appearance to the distal esophagus and mucosal folds (Fig. 11.14). After the evaluation of mucosal pathology, the systematic analysis of the VFE proceeds with an assessment of esophageal motility.

Fig. 11.3 Mucosal irregularities (*red arrowheads*) in a
person with esophageal cancer and a 6-cm stricture of the
cervical esophagus. (Source:
Cardiovasc and Intervent
Radiol 31(3):663–668, 2008)

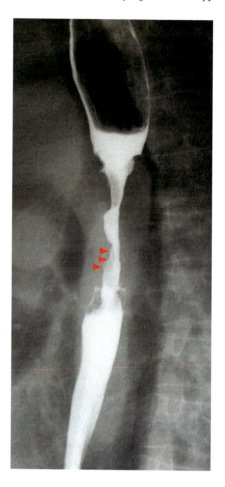

Evaluation of Esophageal Motility

An evaluation of esophageal motility is an essential aspect of the comprehensive
VFE. Motility abnormalities can generally be classified into IEM, esophageal
spasm, scleroderma, or achalasia. IEM is the much more frequent diagnosis. IEM
is further classified on VFE as mild or severe. Motility assessment begins with an
evaluation of primary peristalsis. Primary peristalsis is evaluated by assessing the
primary stripping wave and esophageal stasis. This is initially performed in the upright and then prone position (Chap. 3). It is essential that the patient be instructed to
consume the barium bolus in one effortful swallow. Taking additional swallows will
terminate the esophageal contraction wave and give the impression of dysmotility
when peristalsis is normal (deglutitive inhibition). Primary peristalsis is visualized
fluoroscopically as a stripping wave. A normal esophageal stripping wave transmits a bolus along the esophagus at approximately 2 cm/s. A bolus should clear a

Fig. 11.4 Nodularity of the distal third of the esophagus suggesting the presence of inflammation and reflux esophagitis. (Source: Radiographic Evaluation of the Esophageal Phase of Swallowing Publisher: Springer. Authors: Levine, Marc S. Book title: Manual of Diagnostic and Therapeutic Techniques for Disorders of Deglutition. DOI: 10.1007/978-1-4614-3779-6_4. Published Date: 2013-01-01)

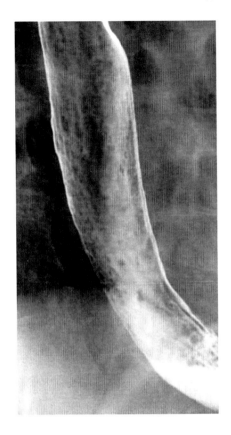

normal 25 cm esophagus in less than 15 s. The barium should proceed throughout its entire length in one smooth stripping motion. The presence of secondary peristalsis is also evaluated. Secondary peristalsis is a contraction that originates in the esophagus as a response to esophageal distention or chemical (acid) stimulation. Secondary peristalsis on VFE is assessed in response to barium stasis within the esophagus. Secondary peristalsis should strip and clear the esophagus of retained barium without the patient initiating a swallow in the pharynx. Barium stasis in the esophagus > 15 s or alterations in the primary or secondary stripping wave are indications of IEM. The degree of peristaltic abnormality is classified as mild, severe (profound), or absent. In patients with profound esophageal dysmotility, it is essential to recognize the presence of **any** stripping wave. A complete absence of a primary and secondary stripping wave suggests achalasia and a complete absence of a stripping wave in the smooth muscle esophagus only (distal 2/3) suggests scleroderma. The visualization of a single primary or secondary stripping wave suggests a diagnosis other than achalasia. The presence of tertiary peristalsis is then evaluated. *Tertiary peristalsis* is simultaneous, isolated, nonperistaltic esophageal contractions (Fig. 6.8 and Fig. 11.15) that occur irrespective of coordinated peristalsis. They are nonpropulsive and are considered a sign of esophageal dysmotility. Profound

Fig. 11.5 Irregular granular esophageal mucosa suggestive of candida esophagitis. (Source: Gastrointestinal Imaging Publisher: Springer Authors: Lee, Susanna I. Thrall, James H. Book title: Choosing the Correct Radiologic Test DOI: 10.1007/978-3-642-15772-1_4 Published Date: 2013-01-01)

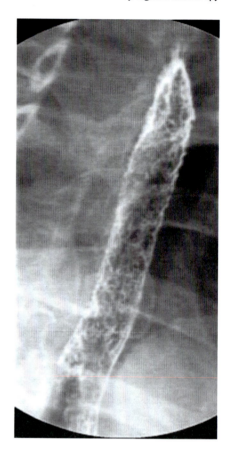

Fig. 11.6 Candida esophagitis seen during esophagoscopy

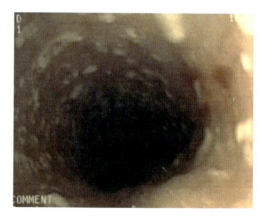

Fig. 11.7 Herpes esophagitis. Multiple small ulcerations, each surrounded by a ring of lucency due to edema, are present in the distal esophagus. (Source: Gastrointestinal infection in the immunocompromised (AIDS) patient Publisher: Springer Authors: Reeders, J. W. A. J. Yee, J. Gore, R. M. Miller, F. H. Megibow, A. J. Journal title: European Radiology Supplements DOI: 10.1007/s00330-003-2065-7 Published Date: 2004-03-01)

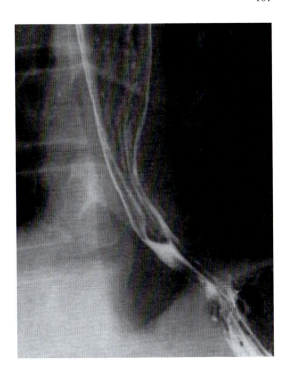

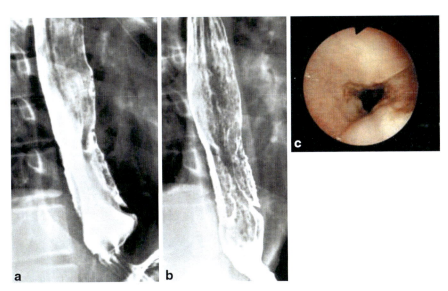

Fig. 11.8 Findings of cytomegalovirus esophagitis include longitudinal, semilunar, deep, penetrating ulcerations at the mid-esophagus opposite each other. a Single-contrast and b double-contrast esophagogram. c Endoscopy. (Source: Gastrointestinal infection in the immunocompromised (AIDS) patient Publisher: Springer Authors: Reeders, J. W. A. J. Yee, J. Gore, R. M. Miller, F. H. Megibow, A. J. Journal title: European Radiology Supplements DOI: 10.1007/s00330-003-2065-7 Published Date: 2004-03-01)

Fig. 11.9 Eosinophilic
esophagitis with ringed
esophagus. There is a
smooth, tapered stricture in
the mid-esophagus with dis-
tinctive ring-like indentations
(*arrows*) in the region of the
stricture. (Source: Radiographic Evaluation of the
Esophageal Phase of Swal-
lowing. Publisher: Springer
Levine, Marc S. Book title:
Manual of Diagnostic and
Therapeutic Techniques for
Disorders of Deglutition.
DOI: 10.1007/978-1-4614-
3779-6_4. Published Date:
2013-01-01)

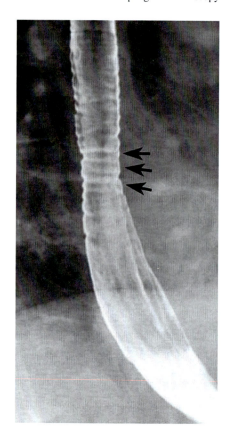

Fig. 11.10 Endoscopic image
of eosinophilic esophagitis
displaying characteristic rings
and giving the appearance of
a corrugated or trachealized
esophagus

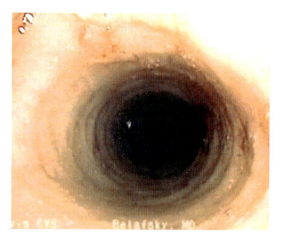

Fig. 11.11 Small-caliber esophagus characteristic of eosinophilic esophagitis

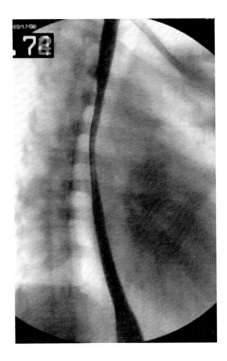

Fig. 11.12 Prominent esophageal mucosal folds (*black arrowheads*) on anterior-posterior fluoroscopic view suggestive of reflux esophagitis

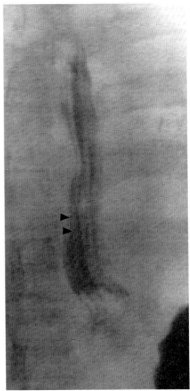

Fig. 11.13 Prominent
esophageal mucosal folds
on esophagoscopy (*black
arrowheads*) indicating reflux
esophagitis

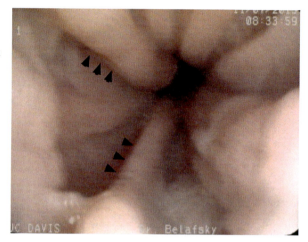

Fig. 11.14 Esophageal varices seen in a prone single-
contrast spot image showing
uphill esophageal varices
as serpiginous longitudinal
defects in the lower esophagus. (Source: Radiographic
Evaluation of the Esopha-
geal Phase of Swallowing
Publisher: Springer. Authors:
Levine, Marc S. Book title:
Manual of Diagnostic and
Therapeutic Techniques for
Disorders of Deglutition.
DOI: 10.1007/978-1-4614-
3779-6_4 Published Date:
2013-01-01)

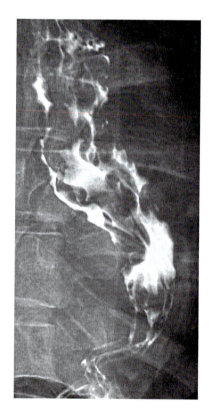

Fig. 11.15 Videofluoroscopic esophagram displaying tertiary contractions
(*black arrows*)

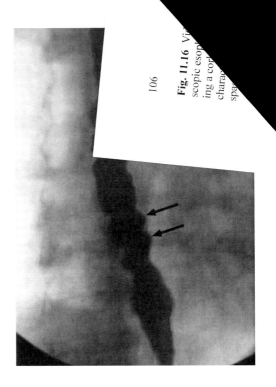

106

Fig. 11.16 Vi
scopic eso
ing a co
chara
spa

tertiary contractions can be seen in esophageal spasm and give the appearance of a
corkscrew esophagus (Figs. 11.16 and 11.17). Tertiary contractions and esophageal
spasm may be associated with underlying gastroesophageal reflux.

After an assessment of primary, secondary, and tertiary peristalsis, the motility
assessment includes an evaluation of stasis and intra-esophageal reflux. Stasis exists
when residual barium remains in the esophagus after the completion of the primary
stripping wave. The entire bolus may cease movement with a failed or dropped
esophageal contraction or the bolus may fragment with an incomplete contraction
with only part of the bolus remaining in the esophagus. The most common location
to visualize barium stasis is in the esophageal dead zone above the aortic compression. This region is a manometric low-pressure zone that exists from the transition
of skeletal to smooth esophageal muscle. The residual barium can be cleared with
a secondary peristaltic wave or can escape proximally. Proximal escape of barium
is termed intra-esophageal reflux and is an indication of esophageal dysmotility not
gastroesophageal reflux disease (GERD). If the barium escapes proximally into the
pharynx it is termed esophago-pharyngeal reflux. After the assessment of peristalsis
and stasis, lower esophageal sphincter (LES) function is evaluated.

The LES should be closed at rest and should relax at the initiation of the pharyngeal swallow. An LES that does not relax adequately suggests constriction (web,
ring, stricture, neoplasm) or a hypertensive LES (incomplete LES relaxation). An
LES that remains open suggests an incompetent LES or scleroderma. An LES that
does not open at all suggests achalasia. Other VFE findings suggestive of achalasia

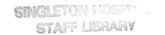

...deofluoro-
...nagram display-
...screw esophagus
...teristic of esophageal
...sm

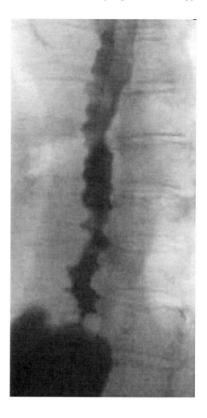

include an atonic, dilated esophagus with the characteristic bird's beak appearance at the distal aspect of the LES (Fig. 11.18). End stage esophageal dilation secondary to achalasia gives the appearance of a large dilated sigmoid esophagus (Fig. 11.19). After the assessment of motility, the analysis of the VFE proceeds with an evaluation of obstructing esophageal pathology.

Evaluation of Obstructing Esophageal Pathology

The entire length of the esophagus is visualized for areas of narrowing. The four normal regions of esophageal compression (PES, aortic arch, left mainstem bronchus, LES) are identified. Administration of a 13 mm barium tablet helps identify luminal narrowing <13 mm. Pharyngoesophageal and cervical esophageal webs are the most common pathology identified. Webs are most common in the region of the PES (Fig. 11.1) but are also seen in the cervical esophagus (Fig. 11.20). The presence of an esophageal ring is then evaluated. The esophageal A-ring demarcates the proximal border of the LES and usually represents normal esophageal anatomy (Fig. 6.11). A-rings can rarely enlarge and produce muscular obstruction

Fig. 11.17 Videofluoroscopic esophagram displaying a corkscrew esophagus
characteristic of esophageal
spasm

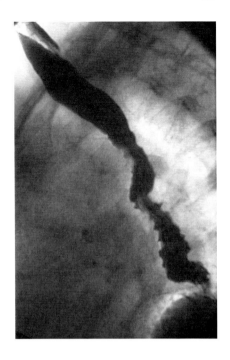

Fig. 11.18 A dilated, atonic
esophagus (*black arrow-
heads*) with the characteristic
birds beak appearance (*black
arrow*) at the distal aspect of
the lower esophageal sphincter representing achalasia.
There is a complete absence
of a primary and secondary
esophageal stripping wave

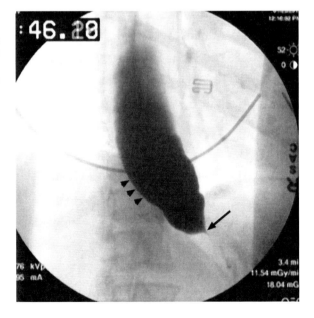

Fig. 11.19 End-stage achalasia. The esophagus is dilated and has a sigmoid appearance (*black arrowheads*) with the characteristic bird's beak appearance (*black arrow*) at the distal aspect of the lower esophageal sphincter. There is a complete absence of a primary and secondary esophageal stripping wave

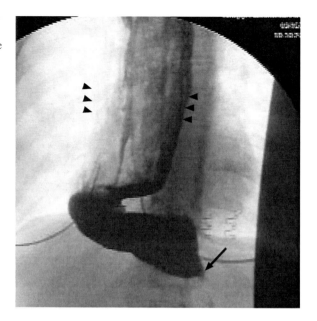

Fig. 11.20 Lateral fluoroscopic view of a cervical esophageal web (*black arrow*). This web is 2 cm distal to the pharyngoesophageal segment and the region of a cricopharyngeal web (Fig. 11.1)

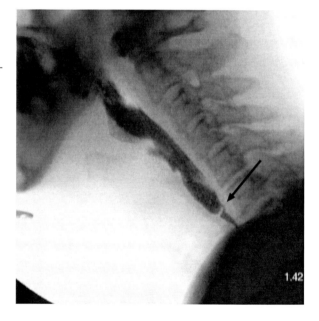

unresponsive to esophageal dilation (Fig. 11.21). The injection of botulinum toxin into an obstructing A-ring may provide symptomatic relief. Schatzki's B-rings are much more common than A-rings. They are fixed mucosal rings that occur at the gastroesophageal junction (GEJ). Although the pathophysiology is uncertain, these

Fig. 11.21 Videofluoroscopic esophagram displaying a constricting esophageal
A ring (**a**) above a dilated
esophageal vestibule (*V*).
Gastric rugae (*small black
arrows*) can be seen migrating above the diaphragm
(*large black arrow*) indicating the presence of a hiatal
hernia. Also seen is a mildly
constricting Schatzki's B
ring (**b**)

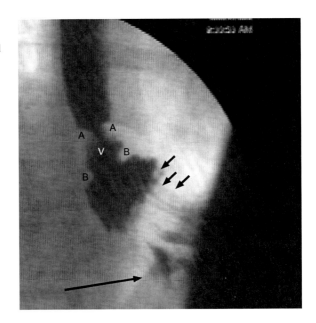

rings are thought to be associated with gastroesophageal reflux. They are a frequent
finding on VFE and may be present in up to 15 % of routine examinations. The
most common presenting symptom of a Schatzki's B-ring is solid food dysphagia.
B-rings, however, are often incidental findings, and comorbid sources of dysphagia such as web, IEM, and esophagitis must be excluded. The luminal narrowing
caused by a B-ring necessary to cause dysphagia is uncertain. Traditional teaching
suggests that luminal narrowing of the esophagus < 13 mm causes the sensation
of dysphagia. This measurement, however, is arbitrary and depends on individual
esophageal sensitivity, comorbid esophageal disease such as esophagitis and ineffective motility, and patient dentition, diet, and chewing habits. Schatzki's B-rings
are located at the GEJ and are usually found in association with a hiatal hernia
(HH) (Figs. 11.22–11.24). The absence of a HH should question the diagnosis of a
Schatzki's B-ring. Large quantities of barium during a sequential swallow task are
necessary to accurately elicit and diagnose both esophageal webs and rings.

Esophageal stricture is the next most common cause of esophageal obstruction.
The most common cause of PES stricture is radiation therapy for head and neck
cancer. The most common cause of esophageal stricture is gastroesophageal reflux
(peptic stricture). Reflux-induced strictures are less common in the era of widespread proton pump inhibitor use (Fig. 11.25). Other significantly less frequent
causes of esophageal stricture include EoE (Fig. 11.9), external beam irradiation
for thoracic tumors (Fig. 11.26), pill- and caustic-induced stenosis (Fig. 11.27),
neoplasm (Fig. 11.28), and Crohn's disease (Fig. 11.29). Stricture from neoplasm
involving the distal esophagus that causes an atonic, dilated esophagus and LES

Fig. 11.22 A Schatzki's B-ring (*black arrows*) on video fluoroscopic esophagram. The ring is at the gastroesophageal junction and is seen in conjunction with a hiatal hernia (*black arrowheads*). *V* esophageal vestibule.

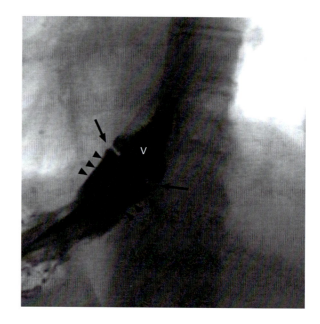

Fig. 11.23 An endoscopic image of a circumferential Schatzki's B-ring (*short black arrows*). Gastric rugae (*black arrowheads*) are extending above the compression caused by the diaphragm (*long black arrow*) indicating the presence of a hiatal hernia. The ring is at the gastroesophageal junction which is identified by the proximal termination of the rugae

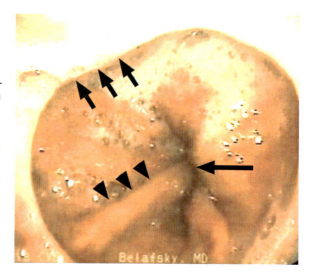

obstruction may cause secondary achalasia (Fig. 11.28). Subtle strictures can be difficult to visualize without distention of the esophagus with the administration of large quantities of barium during the sequential swallow task. Administration of a barium tablet will only identify luminal narrowing < 13 mm.

Vascular anomalies are a rare cause of esophageal obstruction on VFE. The most common vascular causes of dysphagia are a calcified aorta and aortic aneurysm

Fig. 11.24 A Schatzki's
B-ring (*long black arrow*)
on video fluoroscopic
esophagram. There is a small
sliding hiatal hernia (*black
arrowheads*) identified by the
sliding rugae above the diaphragm. Only a small portion
of the gastric cardia is visible
above the diaphragm on this
still image (*proximal black
arrowhead*). Also visible are
tertiary contractions (*short
black arrows*)

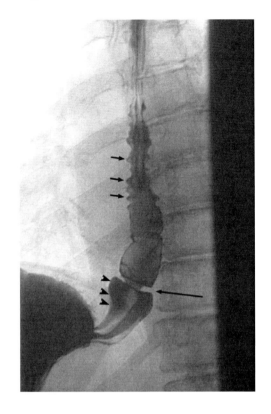

Fig. 11.25 Videofluoroscopic esophagram displaying a peptic stricture (*short
black arrow*) at the gastroesophageal junction. Gastric
rugae can be seen above the
level of the diaphragm (*long
black arrow*) indicating the
presence of a hiatal hernia
(*black arrowheads*)

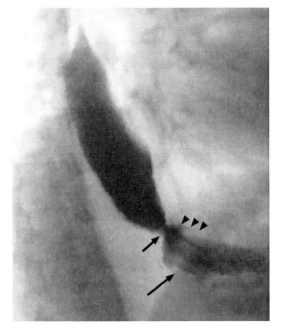

Fig. 11.26 Videofluoroscopic
esophagram displaying a
high-cervical esophageal
stricture secondary to external beam radiation

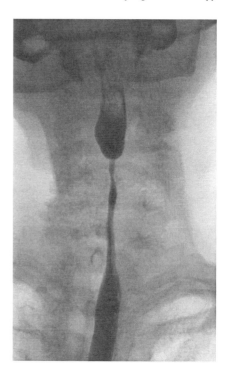

(Fig. 11.30). The next most common vascular cause of dysphagia is an aberrant right
subclavian artery or dysphagia lusoria (Figs. 11.31 and 11.32) followed by a double
aortic arch and a right aortic arch. After the evaluation of obstructing esophageal
pathology the comprehensive VFE proceeds with the identification of diverticuli.

Evaluation of Diverticuli

Hypopharyngeal diverticuli (Zenkers) are much more common than esophageal
diverticuli (Chap. 10). Esophageal diverticuli may be classified as traction and
pulsion diverticuli. Pulsion diverticuli are typically located in the distal esophagus
above the GEJ (epiphrenic) and are associated with IEM and/or a stricture distal
to the diverticula (Fig. 11.33). Small diverticuli may be asymptomatic but large
ones can retain food and liquid and cause dysphagia and regurgitation. Traction

Fig. 11.27 Videofluoroscopic esophagram displaying a long-segment esophageal stricture of the distal half of the esophagus caused by caustic ingestion (lye)

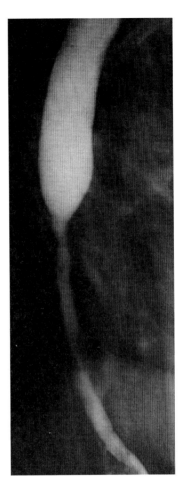

diverticuli occur in the proximal and mid esophagus and are caused by scarring and tethering of the esophagus from tuberculosis, thoracic surgery, fungal infection, and lymphadenopathy (Fig. 11.34). Intramural pseudodiverticula are outpouchings of the esophagus caused by dilated esophageal excretory ducts (Fig. 11.35). They frequently occur in response to an esophageal stricture. The comprehensive VFE proceeds with the identification of HH.

Fig. 11.28 Videofluoroscopic esophagram displaying a stricture at the gastroesophageal junction (*white arrows*) from an invading gastric carcinoma. The mucosa of the lower esophageal sphincter and proximal stomach is irregular and there is a filling defect from retained food in the dilated distal esophagus (*black arrows*). (Source: Radiographic Evaluation of the Esophageal Phase of Swallowing Publisher: Springer Levine, Marc S. Book title: Manual of Diagnostic and Therapeutic Techniques for Disorders of Deglutition DOI: 10.1007/978-1-4614-3779-6_4 Published Date: 2013-01-01)

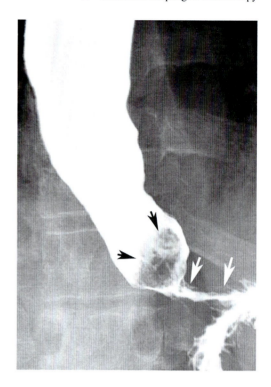

Fig. 11.29 Endoscopic image of a mid-esophageal stricture (*black arrowheads*) from Crohn's disease

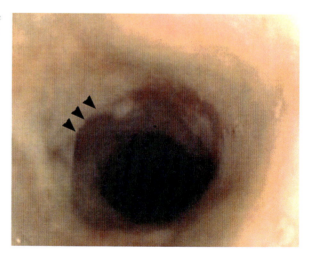

Fig. 11.30 Videofluoro-scopic esophagram display-ing esophageal compression (*black arrowheads*) caused by an aortic aneurysm

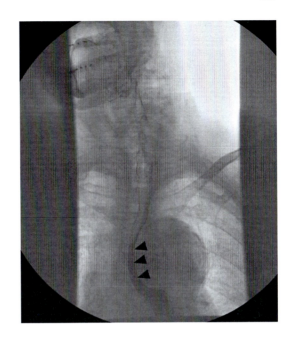

Fig. 11.31 Anatomy of an aberrant right subclavian artery. Right common carotid artery (1), left common carotid artery (2), left subcla-vian artery (3), aberrant right subclavian artery (4), ascend-ing aorta (5), esophagus (6), and left bronchus (7) This lusorian artery is a relatively rare anomaly in which the right subclavian artery arises from the aortic arch distal of the left subclavian artery and crosses the midline behind the esophagus. (Source: Down syndrome and aber-rant right subclavian artery Publisher: Springer Authors: Roofthooft, Marcus T. R. Meer, Hester Rietman, Wim G. Ebels, Tjark Berger, Rolf M. F. Journal title: European Journal of Pediatrics DOI: 10.1007/s00431-007-0637-2 Published Date: 2008-07-16)

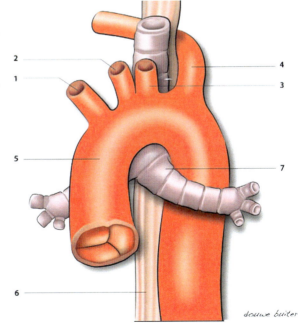

Fig. 11.32 Videofluoroscopic esophagram displaying esophageal compression
caused by an aberrant right
subclavian artery

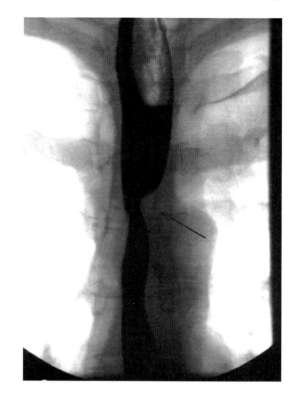

Fig. 11.33 Videofluoroscopic esophagram displaying large pulsion diverticula
(epiphrenic) above the gastroesophageal junction. (Source:
Epiphrenic Diverticulum
of the Esophagus. From
Pathophysiology to Treat-
mentPublisher: Springer
Authors:Soares, Renato Her-
bella, Fernando A. Prachand,
Vivek N. Ferguson, Mark
K. Patti, Marco G. Journal
title: Journal of Gastrointestinal Surgery DOI: 10.1007/
s11605-010-1216-9 Pub-
lished Date: 2010-11-23)

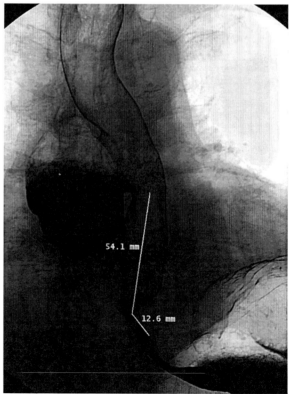

Fig. 11.34 Videofluoro-scopic esophagram display-ing a mid-esophageal traction diverticulum

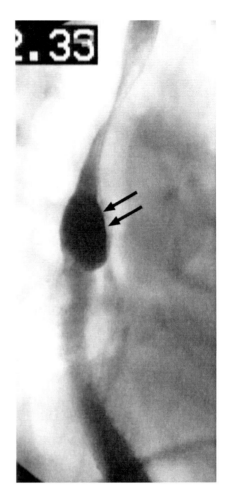

Evaluation of HH

There are four different types of HH classified by the relationship of the GEJ and gastric fundus with the diaphragm (Figs. 11.36–11.43). A type I HH exists when the GEJ has migrated above the diaphragm but the majority of the fundus remains with-in the abdominal cavity (Figs. 11.37 and 11.8). The movement of the distal esopha-gus and gastric cardia is dynamic with the respiratory motion of the diaphragm and the GEJ can slide above the diaphragm and return to its normal anatomical position in the abdomen. Distention of the distal esophagus with large quantities of barium during the sequential swallowing task in the RAO position as well as having the patient perform a Valsalva maneuver is essential to elicit small hernias. Type I HHs are extremely prevalent and may be present in up to 40% of routine VFEs. The majority of patients with a type I HH are asymptomatic but the normal protective

Fig. 11.35 Videofluoroscopic esophagram displaying pseudodiverticulosus
(*white arrows*). (**a**) There
are numerous barium-filled
diverticula of the mid- and
lower esophagus. (**b**) There is
lack of distension of the mid-
esophagus, thus indicating
the presence of a stricture.
(Source: Esophageal intramural pseudodiverticulosis
characterized by barium
esophagography: a case
report Publisher: BioMed
Central Authors: O'Connor,
Owen J Brady, Adrian
Shanahan, Fergus Quigley,
Eamonn O'Riordain, Michael
Maher, Michael M Journal
title: Journal of Medical Case
Reports DOI: 10.1186/1752-
1947-4-145 Published Date:
2010-12-01)

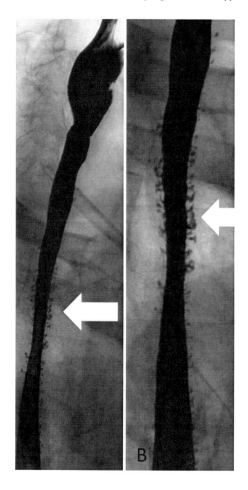

Fig. 11.36 Diagram of the
normal anatomic relationship
of the gastroesophageal junction (GEJ). The GEJ remains
at or below the level of the
diaphragm. The Angle of HIS
(A) is intact and maintains its
contribution to reflux protection. *E* esophagus

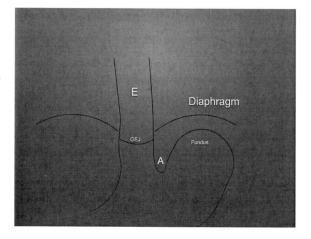

Fig. 11.37 Diagram of a type I (sliding) hiatal hernia (HH). The gastroesophageal junction (GEJ) has migrated above the diaphragm into the chest. The Angle of HIS (A) is blunted, reducing its ability to protect against gastroesophageal reflux

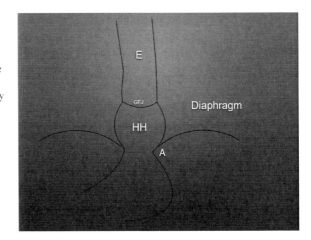

Fig. 11.38 Videofluoroscopic esophagram displaying a type I (sliding) hiatal hernia. The gastric rugae can be seen migrating above the diaphragm (*short black arrow*) to form the hernia (*black arrowheads*). There is a constricting Schatzki's B-ring (*long black arrow*) immediately proximal to the hernia and a slight compression from the esophageal A-ring (*white arrow*) immediately proximal to the mildly dilated vestibule (V). Also visible are moderate tertiary contractions (TC)

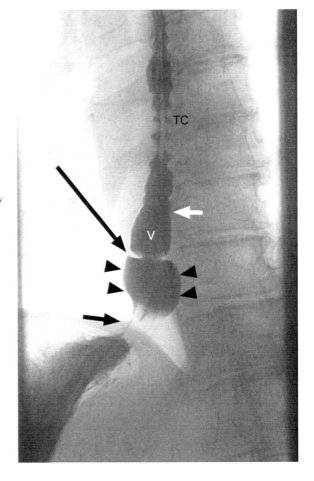

Fig. 11.39 Diagram of a type II hiatal hernia. A type II hernia is a pure paraesophageal hiatal hernia (PEHH) and the gastroesophageal junction (GEJ) remains at or below the level of the diaphragm

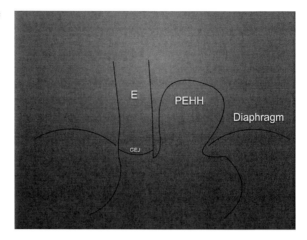

Fig. 11.40 Videofluoroscopic esophagram displaying a type II hiatal hernia. The gastroesophageal junction is at the level of the diaphragm (*long black arrow*) and the gastric fundus has migrated above the GEJ into the chest to form the hernia (*black arrowheads*)

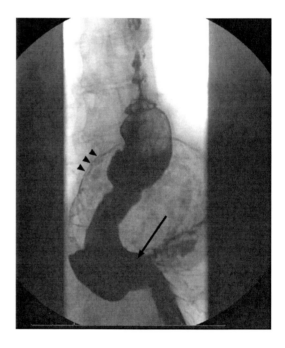

barrier of the LES is diminished and patients with a type I HH are predisposed to experience symptoms related to GERD such as heartburn and regurgitation. A type II HH is a true paraesophageal HH. The GEJ remains within the abdominal cavity at or below the level of the diaphragm. The fundus has migrated above the diaphragm into the chest (Figs. 11.39 and 11.40). A type III HH is a mixed hernia in which the fundus and GEJ have migrated alongside each other above the diaphragm into the

Fig. 11.41 Diagram of a
type III (mixed) hiatal hernia
(MHH). A type III hiatal
hernia is a mixed hernia in
which the fundus and gastroesophageal junction (GEJ)
have herniated alongside each
other above the diaphragm
into the chest. The majority of paraesophageal hiatal
hernias are type III

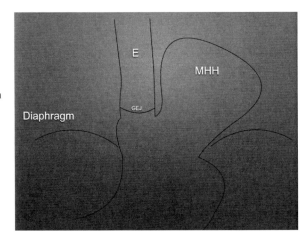

Fig. 11.42 Videofluoroscopic esophagram displaying a type III mixed hiatal
hernia. The gastroesophageal
junction (*short black arrow*)
has migrated with the fundus
(*black arrowheads*) above
the diaphragm (*long black
arrow*) into the chest

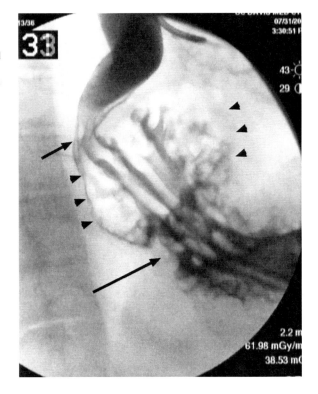

chest (Figs. 11.41 and 11.42). The majority of paraesophageal HHs are mixed type
III. A type IV HH exists when other organs (colon, small intestine, spleen) migrate
with the fundus into the chest (Fig. 11.43). After the evaluation of HH, the VFE
concludes with the assessment of gastroesophageal reflux.

Fig. 11.43 Videofluoroscopic esophagram displaying a type IV mixed hiatal
hernia

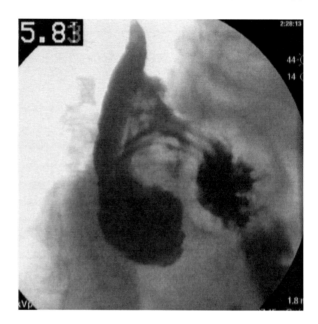

Evaluation of Gastroesophageal Reflux

The VFE is poorly sensitive and specific for the diagnosis of GERD. Estimates of
its sensitivity may be as low as 20 %. The fluoroscopic examination is only able to
detect the regurgitation of barium from the stomach into the esophagus. We differentiate the presence of barium regurgitation (BR) during the VFE from a diagnosis
of GERD. BR is a fluoroscopic finding and not a criterion for disease diagnosis. The
presence of BR during the examination does not ensure that a patient's symptoms
are due to GERD and the absence of BR does not exclude GERD as a cause of a
patient's symptoms. Nonetheless, the presence of BR on VFE within the context
of other fluoroscopic findings such as IEM and HH can add to the overall clinical picture and help formulate treatment recommendations. The presence of BR is
evaluated with the patient in the supine position. A pillow is placed under the head
to simulate nocturnal positioning and provocative maneuvers such as a leg raise,
Valsalva maneuver, and water siphon test are performed (Chap. 3). BR on VFE is
classified as trace, moderate, and severe (Fig. 11.44). BR from the stomach into the
esophagus is also differentiated from intra-esophageal reflux and esophago-pharyngeal reflux, which are both findings suggestive of IEM.

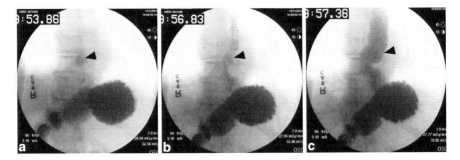

Fig. 11.44 Videofluoroscopic esophagram displaying sequential images of severe gastroesophageal reflux. There is trace (**a**), then moderate (**b**), then profound (**c**) regurgitation of barium all the way to the proximal esophagus

Suggested Reading

Levine MS, Rubesin SE. Diseases of the esophagus: diagnosis with esophagography. Radiology. 2005 Nov;237(2):414–27.

Pickhardt PJ, Arluk GM, editors. Atlas of gastrointestinal imaging. Philadelphia: Saunders; 2007.

Richter J, Castell D, editors. The esophagus. 5th edn. Oxford: Wiley-Blackwell; 2012.

Shaker R, Belafsky PC, Postma GN, Easterling C, editors. Principles of deglutition: a multidisciplinary text for swallowing and its disorders. New York: Springer; 2012.

Shaker R, Belafsky PC, Postma GN, Easterling C, editors. Manual of diagnostic and therapeutic techniques for disorders of deglutition. New York: Springer; 2012.

Index

P. C. Belafsky, M. A. Kuhn, *The Clinician's Guide to Swallowing Fluoroscopy,*
DOI 10.1007/978-1-4939-1109-7, © Springer Science+Business Media New York 2014

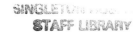

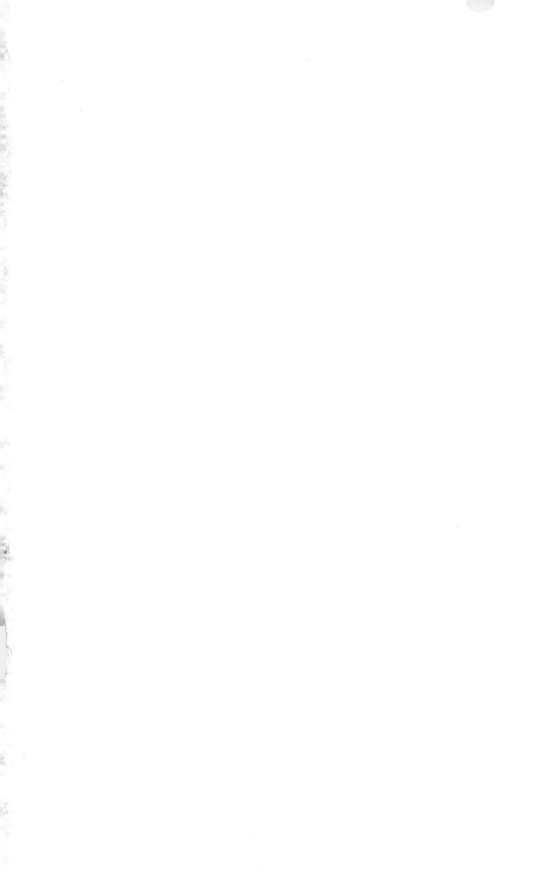

Printed by Books on Demand, Germany